the anti-inflammatory recipe book

Relieve symptoms of gut disorders, chronic pain and autoimmune diseases with over 100 fresh and nutritious recipes

Angela Dowden

Registered Nutritionist

First published in Great Britain in 2025
by Hamlyn, an imprint of
Octopus Publishing Group Ltd
Carmelite House
50 Victoria Embankment
London EC4Y 0DZ
www.octopusbooks.co.uk

An Hachette UK Company
www.hachette.co.uk

Some of this material has previously appeared in Hamlyn All Colour *200 Juice Diet Recipes, 200 Healthy Feasts, 200 Easy Vegetarian Dishes, 200 Veggie Feasts, 200 Vegan Feasts, 200 Gluten-free Recipes, 200 Light Gluten-free Recipes and 200 Super Salads.*

The authorised representative in the EEA is Hachette Ireland,
8 Castlecourt Centre,
Castleknock Road,
Castleknock, Dublin 15,
D15 YF6A, Ireland

Text copyright © Octopus Publishing Group Ltd 2025

Distributed in the US by
Hachette Book Group
1290 Avenue of the Americas,
4th and 5th Floors
New York, NY 10104

Distributed in Canada by Canadian Manda Group, 664 Annette St., Toronto, Ontario, Canada M6S 2C8

All rights reserved. No part of this work may be reproduced or utilized in any form or by any means, electronic or mechanical, including photocopying, recording or by any information storage and retrieval system, without the prior written permission of the publisher.

ISBN 978 0 60063 868 1

A CIP catalogue record for this book is available from the British Library.

Printed and bound in China.

10 9 8 7 6 5 4 3 2 1

Commissioning Editor:
　Louisa Johnson
Photographers: Frank Adam,
　Stephen Conroy, Will Heap,
　David Munns, Lis Parsons,
　William Shaw and Ian Wallace
Art director: Jaz Bahra
Project Editor: Vicky Orchard
Deputy Picture Manager: Jennifer Veal
Production Manager: Lucy Carter and
　Nic Jones

Cookery notes
Standard level spoon measurement are used in all recipes.
1 tablespoon – one 15 ml spoon
1 teaspoon – one 5 ml spoon

Both imperial and metric measurements have been given in all recipes. Use one set of measurements only and not a mixture of both.

Eggs should be medium unless otherwise stated.

Fresh herbs should be used unless otherwise stated. If unavailable use dried herbs as an alternative but halve the quantities stated.

Pepper should be freshly ground black pepper unless otherwise stated.

> All reasonable care has been taken in the preparation of this book but the information it contains is not intended to take the place of treatment by a qualified medical practitioner. Before making any changes in your health regime, always consult a doctor. Any application of the ideas and information contained in this book is at the reader's sole discretion and risk.

Contents

Introduction	4
Meal Plans	13
Breakfast	18
Salads & Leafy Greens	48
Snacks & Starters	86
Main Meals to Heal	120
Light Bites & Sides	158
Something Sweet	192
Index	220
Glossary	224
Picture Credits	224

Introduction

As we learn more about chronic inflammation and its impact on our bodies, the importance of an anti-inflammatory diet is becoming increasingly clear. Inflammation is connected to a range of serious health problems, including heart disease, diabetes and dementia. Our daily food choices can either fuel persistent inflammation and increase the potential for disease or help to reduce it, creating better health and wellbeing.

While there is no one specific anti-inflammatory diet, an eating plan that quells inflammation tends to be rich in vitamins and minerals, low in highly processed and sugary foods and largely plant based. A Mediterranean-style diet is a good example.

On the other hand, a pro-inflammatory diet typically includes high amounts of ultra-processed foods, sugars and animal fats, and is characterized by overeating and a lack of essential nutrients. The Western-style diet, which is now the norm in the UK and the USA is a classic example.

Transitioning to an anti-inflammatory diet requires commitment but is also enjoyable. Eating this way cuts a lot of the 'boring beige' from your diet, replacing it with vibrant colours and textures. It also doesn't mean eliminating all treats – plain dark chocolate, for instance, can still have a place in this diet.

While reducing your risk of future diseases may be your primary motivation for adopting an anti-inflammatory diet, you may also enjoy immediate health benefits, such as increased energy levels and enhanced mood, which can strengthen your resolve to stay on track.

To keep you inspired, the recipes in the following chapters are designed to be simple, enjoyable and bursting with flavour. Coupled with a four-week meal planner and a comprehensive guide to inflammation-fighting ingredients, *The Anti-Inflammatory Recipe Book* gives you all the tools you need to create menus that combat inflammation and ill health, and make you feel great.

How chronic inflammation creates harm

Acute, or short-term Inflammation – characterized by the swelling and redness you get around a wound, for example – is a key part of how our body protects and heals itself. It's the process whereby blood flow and immune activity in the area increase, fighting off harmful things like bacteria, viruses or injuries. When inflammation stays contained, tissues get repaired, and everything gets back to normal.

However, chronic Inflammation, which is the harmful type, is when lower-grade inflammation lasts for a long time. This is often due to continuous exposure to harmful triggers like free radicals and oxidative stress (caused by things like poor diet, smoking and pollution), or persistent infections. Obesity is another factor that increases inflammation, and up to 3 per cent of people also carry a gene variant that may increase their inflammation risk.[1]

When inflammation continues, it can lead to long-term damage in various organs and tissues, contributing to many diseases. The symptoms and effects can vary depending on which part of the body is affected and what's causing the inflammation.

Chronic inflammation often starts in your gut

Scientists have discovered that inflammation often starts with the microbiome – the huge collection of microbes living within our intestines.[2] The gut microbiome interacts with the many immune cells in the gut, helping to teach our body to distinguish between harmless bacteria and harmful invaders.

Specific microbes within our gut can influence decisions about which cells to destroy or let live by activating immune components that either promote or suppress inflammation. When the microbiome–immune system relationship works well, inflammation is kept under control. However, when there are too many pro-inflammatory immune cells or not enough anti-inflammatory ones to balance them out, things can go wrong.

Problems with the microbiome might cause the immune system to mistakenly attack healthy tissue, thereby playing a major role in various inflammatory conditions inside the gut and beyond. One of the key features of an anti-inflammatory diet is being able to support the health of the microbiome.

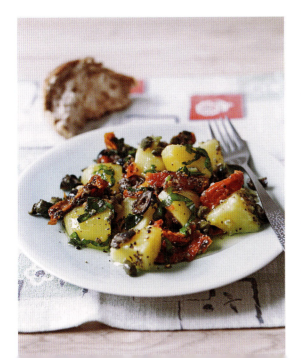

Inflammation, diets and disease

Eating more healthily can help guard against or ease a variety of health conditions that are related to chronic inflammation in the body. These are some of the inflammatory conditions that an anti-inflammatory diet can help:

Cardiovascular disease

Chronic inflammation in the blood vessels can contribute to atherosclerosis and high blood pressure, which in turn increases the risk of having a heart attack or a stroke.

A large US-based study which looked at 210,145 women and men over 32 years found that participants whose diets had higher inflammatory potential were at greater risk of cardiovascular disease. After taking into account the use of anti-inflammatory medications and other risk factors, it showed those with the most inflammatory diets had a 46 per cent higher risk of coronary heart disease and a 28 per cent higher risk of stroke.[3]

Conversely, the research confirmed that people who consumed diets high in anti-inflammatory foods had a lower risk of developing cardiovascular disease.

Cancer

Over time, chronic inflammation can cause DNA damage and lead to cancer. For example, people with inflammatory bowel disease are at increased risk of colon cancer.

One analysis of 44 individual studies found that each increase in dietary inflammatory index score (see pages 7–8), was associated with an 8 per cent increase in overall cancer risk, with colorectal cancer being the most strongly linked with inflammation.[4]

An anti-inflammatory diet can also work in ways beyond controlling inflammation to reduce cancer risk. For example, the phytonutrients and antioxidants it contains play a role in cancer-preventative pathways, including carcinogen deactivation, cell-to-cell signalling and destruction of abnormal cells.

Neurocognitive decline
Inflammation in the brain is thought to be behind cognitive decline, while anti-inflammatory diets, like the Mediterranean diet, have been associated with significant reductions in the incidence of Alzheimer's disease and other forms of dementia.[5, 6]

The PREDIMED study found that an anti-inflammatory Mediterranean diet can positively impact brain function when followed long term. Older adults who followed this diet for 4–6 years showed better cognitive function, including improved thinking skills, memory and decision-making abilities, compared to those on a control diet.[7]

Some research also suggests that an anti-inflammatory diet may reduce the risk of Parkinson's disease and help manage the condition.[8]

Type 2 diabetes
Chronic inflammation can predispose people to type 2 diabetes as it contributes to insulin resistance, a condition in which the body does not respond effectively to insulin (the hormone that regulates blood sugar levels). Elevated insulin levels can exacerbate inflammation, further worsening insulin resistance and perpetuating the cycle.

One study found that people who ate an anti-inflammatory diet were 29 per cent less likely to develop diabetes if they started with normal blood

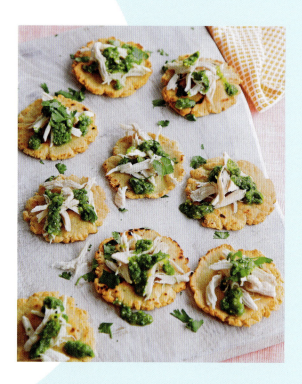

sugar levels. For those who already had slightly high blood sugar levels (prediabetes), their risk of developing diabetes was 19 per cent lower.[9]

Arthritis
Most types of arthritis involve inflammation. Rheumatoid arthritis specifically is an autoimmune condition (the immune system attacks the joints), and may be particularly responsive to an anti-inflammatory diet.

In a 2021 review and meta-analysis of 19 different trials, people with rheumatoid arthritis who ate anti-inflammatory diets reported significantly less pain compared to those on regular diets. Longer studies (lasting three months or more) tended to show more significant pain reduction and people with higher bodyweight saw greater pain improvements that were not directly linked to weight loss.[10]

It should be stated, however, that these studies were hard to compare and had potentially biased results, so more and better research is needed.

Metabolic syndrome

Inflammation can impair fat and glucose metabolism and increase oxidation, contributing to the cluster of conditions known as metabolic syndrome. Typical signs of metabolic syndrome include high blood pressure, high blood sugar, excess abdominal fat, and unhealthy cholesterol and triglyceride levels.

A study that used data from America's National Health and Nutrition Examination Survey (NHANES), involving over 8,000 participants, found that people with the most inflammatory diets were about 1.6 times more likely to have metabolic syndrome compared to those with the least inflammatory diets.[11]

People who ate a lot of anti-inflammatory foods had significantly better metabolic health indicators, including smaller waist circumference, lower triglycerides and lower blood pressure.

Obesity contributes to inflammation and vice versa

Carrying excess fat, especially around the abdomen, can ramp up inflammation. This is because fat tissue releases molecules known as cytokines, which signal to the immune system that the body is under attack.

Part of the immune system's response to obesity is to increase inflammation levels, but the relationship is bidirectional; increased inflammation can also contribute to further fat gain.

Some of the mechanisms whereby inflammation contributes to obesity include those already discussed, such as insulin resistance and impaired fat and sugar metabolism. Inflammatory signals can also affect the brain's regulation of hunger and energy balance, leading to increased appetite.

Fortunately, weight loss can reduce inflammation and even modest weight loss can help.[12] Studies have shown that a 5–10 per cent reduction in bodyweight can also lower inflammation-driven illnesses like metabolic syndrome.[13]

Increasing exercise, being mindful of portion sizes and following an anti-inflammatory diet can help you achieve this small reduction in weight and start to reverse the inflammatory cycle.

Foods that influence inflammation

We have extensive data on pro- and anti-inflammatory foods and nutrients, thanks to a tool called the Dietary Inflammatory Index (DII).

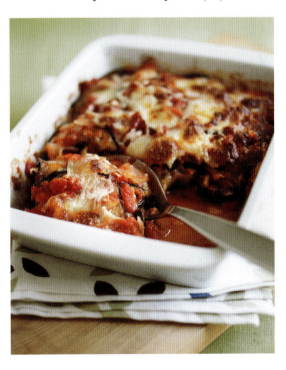

Developed from a vast collection of data exploring the impact of diet on inflammatory markers in the body, the DII assigns positive numeric scores to foods that increase inflammation and negative scores to those that decrease it.

For researchers, the DII represents a standardized method to assess the inflammatory potential of a diet. For you and me, it provides valuable insights into what we should consume more or less of to manage inflammation and reduce our risk of developing inflammatory conditions.

Inflammatory foods

According to the dietary inflammatory index, components that can increase inflammation include:

- Fatty foods, especially those high in saturated fats, trans fats and omega-6 fatty acids.
  – Processed meats like sausages, hot dogs, bacon, salami, chorizo
  – Fried and takeaway foods such as French fries, fried chicken, doughnuts and crisps
  – High-fat dairy foods including cream, crème fraîche, cheese and butter

- Refined (fast-releasing) carbohydrates and added sugars.
  – Soft-textured white breads and pastries, cakes, desserts, chocolate bars, sweets and other sugary snacks
  – Sugar-sweetened beverages like energy drinks, cola and some other fizzy drinks

- Salty (high sodium foods)
  – Processed foods that have more than 1.5 g salt (600 mg sodium) per 100 g or per portion

- Alcoholic drinks, especially spirits
  – Whisky, vodka, gin and brandy

Consuming excess calories and rapid weight gain can also lead to inflammation as the body assumes that the excess fat is a form of 'injury' that requires an immune response.

Anti-inflammatory foods

Foods and nutrients that are anti-inflammatory according to the Dietary Inflammatory Index include:

- Vegetables and fruit rich in antioxidants (flavonoids, beta-carotene and vitamin C), e.g.
  – Leafy green vegetables like spinach, kale, broccoli, asparagus, rocket and watercress
  – Orange/red fruit and veg such as peppers, squashes, tomatoes and apricots
  – Berries such as blueberries, strawberries and raspberries
  – Citrus fruits such as lemons and oranges

- Foods rich in omega-3 fatty acids, monounsaturates and the fat-soluble antioxidant vitamin E, e.g.
  – Oily fish such as salmon, mackerel and sardines (canned and fresh)
  – Nuts and seeds, particularly walnuts, almonds, hazelnuts, flaxseeds and chia seeds
  – Olive oil and rapeseed oil

- Fresh and dried herbs and spices, including
  – Turmeric
  – Ginger
  – Rosemary
  – Black pepper

- Garlic, onions and leeks

- High-fibre plant foods, including many of the fruits and veg above, as well soy-based foods like tofu, pulses and whole grains

- Tea, especially green tea, coffee and cocoa

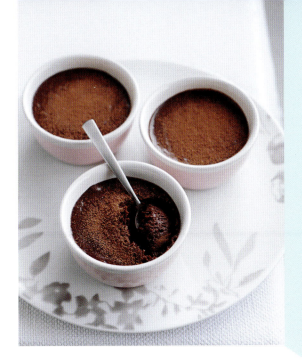

Magnesium (good sources include leafy greens, Brazil nuts, and whole grains), vitamin D (the sunshine vitamin), and several B vitamins (adequately supplied by any well-balanced diet) are also noted by the DII as being anti-inflammatory.

Fermented foods like kefir, sauerkraut, kimchi and kombucha are also considered beneficial for reducing inflammation and supporting overall health. This is because of their positive impact on the gut microbiome.

Neutral foods

Some foods don't influence inflammation very much, or they span the spectrum from mildly anti-inflammatory to mildly inflammatory depending on how much you eat and your individual metabolic response.

- Lean meats like poultry and modest portions of unprocessed red meat are generally neutral.

- Whole or only lightly processed starchy carbs (including all types of pasta, brown rice, skin-on potatoes, lentils, chickpeas, and wholegrain, sourdough or seeded breads), have a neutral effect or are mildly anti-inflammatory. However, if your portions are too large, or you don't metabolize carbs very well, they may switch to being inflammatory.

- Cheese and other high-fat dairy products are generally inflammatory, but low-fat dairy products like semi-skimmed milk, natural yogurt and kefir are neutral or mildly anti-inflammatory.

- Plant-based proteins like tofu are generally anti-inflammatory due to their high antioxidant and low saturated fat content, but vegan 'fake' meats, for example, or burgers that 'bleed' are highly processed and less likely to be anti-inflammatory.

- Alcoholic drinks are inflammatory, but one small glass of red wine with a meal might be the exception because of the antioxidants in red grapes.

- Fruit juice contains a lot of free sugars, but also supplies vitamin C, so one small glass daily can be included in an anti-inflammatory eating plan.

What about gluten?

Gluten can be neutral or inflammatory depending on your body's ability to process it. Most people can consume gluten without experiencing any inflammatory response. However, individuals with coeliac disease must strictly avoid gluten.

Some people have milder sensitivities to gluten – if this applies to you, it's a good idea to minimize your gluten intake to avoid increasing your inflammatory load.

What about additives?

Additives like sweeteners, emulsifiers and preservatives are often said to be inflammatory, but we don't have enough information to say for sure. It may just be that these additives are more commonly found in unhealthy ultra-processed foods, rather than causing inflammation directly.

That said, some evidence suggests that certain emulsifiers and sweeteners may affect the gut microbiome and indirectly contribute to inflammation. By choosing more whole foods and fewer ultra-processed options, you naturally consume fewer additives anyway.

There's no need to meticulously check every label, as a few additives here and there are unlikely to have a significant impact within the context of your overall anti-inflammatory diet.

Chocolate can be part of an anti-inflammatory diet

Chocolate, specifically plain dark chocolate with a high cocoa content (70 per cent or above), is generally considered to have anti-inflammatory properties, despite the fact it also contains saturated fat and sugar. The main reason is its high flavanol content, which are a type of flavonoid with antioxidant and anti-inflammatory effects found in cocoa beans.

In one recent meta-analysis of 33 chocolate and cocoa studies, researchers concluded that plain dark chocolate and cocoa helped lower levels of C-reactive protein (CRP), a marker in the blood that indicates inflammation. Additionally, high-cocoa chocolate mitigated oxidative stress, which causes cellular damage, and enhanced nitric oxide production, helping to improve blood flow.[14]

9 simple ways to make your diet more anti-inflammatory

1. **Eat more fruits and vegetables:** Incorporate a variety of colours.

2. **Choose whole grains:** Opt for brown rice, quinoa, and wholemeal bread over white bread and white rice.

3. **Include healthy fats:** Especially omega-3-rich oily fish and monounsaturate-rich olive oil.

4. **Limit ultra-processed foods:** Cook for yourself rather than using pre-packaged food as often as possible.

5. **Enjoy plain dark chocolate:** Treat yourself to dark chocolate with at least 70 per cent cocoa content.

6. **Incorporate spices and herbs:** Especially turmeric, ginger and garlic.

7. **Drink green tea:** Swap sugary beverages for green tea (black tea and coffee are good, too).

8. **Reduce processed meat intake:** Choose lean unprocessed protein sources like fish, poultry, lean red meat (in moderation) and plant-based proteins such as tofu and legumes.

9. **Moderate alcohol consumption:** If you drink alcohol, do so only in moderation and choose red wine.

A note on these recipes

When aiming to reduce your inflammation, what matters most is your overall pattern of eating rather than individual dishes.

That's why in this book, you'll find a variety of recipes that cater to both health and enjoyment. While not every ingredient in every recipe is strictly anti-inflammatory, we believe in a holistic approach to dietary health. This means balancing nutrient-rich ingredients with occasional indulgences to create an enjoyable, sustainable diet that promotes anti-inflammatory benefits.

Obviously, if you only ever used recipes from the sweets chapter, it wouldn't achieve a balanced anti-inflammatory diet. But by selecting recipes from all the chapters, you'll lower inflammation, increase your overall wellbeing and feel great.

For extra guidance, the following four-week menu will help you get off to a flying start.

Other lifestyle changes that will reduce inflammation

Changing your diet and using the recipes and eating plan in this book can be helpful in reducing inflammation. But dietary measures work best alongside an anti-inflammatory lifestyle, which entails being active, sleeping well and managing stress.

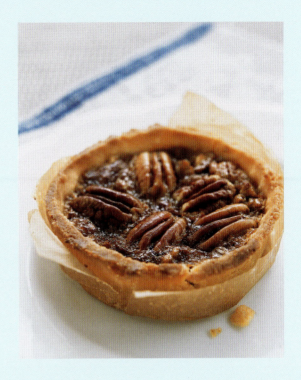

Exercise

People who engage in regular physical activity tend to have lower levels of inflammation, In fact, inflammation markers drop after just one 20-minute stint on a treadmill according to research.[15] Consistency is key and you should aim to do:

- 150 minutes of moderate-intensity aerobic activity per week, such as brisk walking (or 75 minutes of vigorous-intensity activity per week, such as running).

- Two sessions of muscle-strengthening activities, like weightlifting or using resistance bands, per week.

Get enough quality sleep

Sleep helps the body heal and repair, and regulates essential hormones. When you get insufficient or poor-quality sleep, inflammation levels increase and your risk of associated conditions like type 2 diabetes and weight gain also increase.

- Aim for 7 hours of restful sleep per night.

- Follow healthy sleep hygiene habits like maintaining a regular bedtime and waking time, not having phones or iPads by the bed and having a wind-down routine before getting into bed.

Manage stress

Chronic stress, whether physical, mental or emotional, can increase inflammation. The previous steps – being active and getting good-quality sleep – will support stress management, but some additional techniques to try include:

- Mindfulness meditations (using an app to guide you through meditations can be helpful for beginners)

- Simple deep-breathing exercises

- Yoga

- T'ai chi

Bibliography

1. Garnish, S.E., Martin, K.R., Kauppi M., Jackson, V.E., Ambrose, R., Eng, V.V., et al., 'A common human MLKL polymorphism confers resistance to negative regulation by phosphorylation', *Nat Commun.* (2023); Sep 28; 14(1): 6046.

2. Al Bander, Z., Nitert, M.D., Mousa, A., Naderpoor, N., 'The gut microbiota and inflammation: an overview', *Int J Environ Res Public Health.* (2020); Oct 19; 17(20).

3. Li, J., Lee, D.H., Hu, J., Tabung, F.K., Li, Y., Bhupathiraju, S.N., et al., 'Dietary inflammatory potential and risk of cardiovascular disease among men and women in the U.S', *J Am Coll Cardiol.* (2020); Nov 10; 76(19): 2181–93.

4. Li, D., Hao, X., Li, J., Wu, Z., Chen, S., Lin, J., et al., 'Dose-response relation between dietary inflammatory index and human cancer risk: evidence from 44 epidemiologic studies involving 1,082,092 participants', *Am J Clin Nutr.* (2018); Mar 1; 107(3): 371–88.

5. Singh, B., Parsaik, A.K., Mielke, M.M., Erwin, P.J., Knopman, D.S., Petersen, R.C., et al., 'Association of mediterranean diet with mild cognitive impairment and Alzheimer's disease: a systematic review and meta-analysis', *J Alzheimers Dis.* (2014); 39(2): 271–82.

6. Charisis, S., Ntanasi, E., Yannakoulia, M., Anastasiou, C.A., Kosmidis, M.H., Dardiotis, E., et al., 'Mediterranean diet and risk for dementia and cognitive decline in a Mediterranean population', *J Am Geriatr Soc.* (2021); Jun; 69(6): 1548–59.

7. Valls-Pedret, C., Sala-Vila, A., Serra-Mir, M., Corella, D., de la Torre, R., Martínez-González, M.Á., et al., 'Mediterranean Diet and Age-Related Cognitive Decline: A Randomized Clinical Trial', *JAMA Intern Med.* (2015); Jul; 175(7): 1094–103.

8. Zeng, Z., Cen, Y., Wang, L., Luo, X., 'Association between dietary inflammatory index and Parkinson's disease from National Health and Nutrition Examination Survey (2003–2018): a cross-sectional study', *Front Neurosci.* (2023); Jul 20; 17:1203979.

9. Yang, R., Lin, J., Yang, H., Dunk, M.M., Wang, J., Xu, W., et al., 'A low-inflammatory diet is associated with a lower incidence of diabetes: role of diabetes-related genetic risk', *BMC Med.* (2023); Dec 5; 21(1): 483.

10. Schönenberger, K.A., Schüpfer, A-C., Gloy, V.L., Hasler, P., Stanga, Z., Kaegi-Braun, N., et al., 'Effect of Anti-Inflammatory Diets on Pain in Rheumatoid Arthritis: A Systematic Review and Meta-Analysis', *Nutrients.* (2021); Nov 24; 13(12).

11. Zhang, X., Guo, Y., Yao, N., Wang, L., Sun, M., Xu, X., et al., 'Association between dietary inflammatory index and metabolic syndrome: Analysis of the NHANES 2005–2016', *Front Nutr.* (2022); Oct 6; 9: 991907.

12. Bianchi, V.E., 'Weight loss is a critical factor to reduce inflammation', *Clin Nutr ESPEN.* (2018); Dec; 28:21–35.

13. Knell, G., Li, Q., Pettee Gabriel, K., Shuval, K., 'Long-Term Weight Loss and Metabolic Health in Adults Concerned With Maintaining or Losing Weight: Findings From NHANES', *Mayo Clin Proc.* (2018); Nov; 93(11): 1611–6.

14. Behzadi, M., Bideshki, M.V., Ahmadi-Khorram, M., Zarezadeh, M., Hatami, A., 'Effect of dark chocolate/ cocoa consumption on oxidative stress and inflammation in adults: A GRADE-assessed systematic review and dose-response meta-analysis of controlled trials', *Complement Ther Med.* (2024); Jun 24; 84: 103061.

15. Dimitrov, S., Hulteng, E., Hong, S., 'Inflammation and exercise: Inhibition of monocytic intracellular TNF production by acute exercise via β2-adrenergic activation', *Brain Behav Immun.* (2017); Mar; 61:60–8.

Meal Plans

Here you will find four anti-inflammatory weekly meal plans to get you started. Your main meals should include at least 2–3 portions of vegetables or salad, so add extra where necessary. One portion consists of about 3 heaped tablespoons of cooked veg or a bowlful of mixed salad.

To drink, have tea (especially green tea), herbal teas, coffee (though not if caffeine sensitive), and water.

Week one

	BREAKFAST	LUNCH	DINNER	SNACKS
MONDAY	Porridge with semi-skimmed milk, topped with frozen mixed berries (thawed) and a heaped teaspoon nut butter and a drizzle of honey	Watermelon, feta & herb salad (see page 62)	Vegetable 'paella' with almonds (see page 146)	Heaped tablespoon of Harissa & tahini hummus (see page 102) served with carrot and cucumber sticks
TUESDAY	Homemade muesli (see page 42) served with with natural yogurt and a handful of blueberries and strawberries	Cannellini & green bean salad (see page 54)	Garlic & tomato seafood spaghetti (see page 145)	Handful of walnuts; 2 clementines
WEDNESDAY	Florentine-style eggs (see page 45); 150 ml (¼ pint) glass orange juice	Ciabatta toasties with Mediterranean vegetables (see page 174)	Crusted salmon with tomato salsa (see page 149)	2 pea & mint falafels with mint dip (see page 98)
THURSDAY	Fruit granola bars (see page 36); bowl of mixed berries	Baked sweet potato topped with crumbled feta, rocket and a drizzle of lemon-flavoured olive oil	Chicken, lemon & olive stew (see page 142)	Heaped tablespoon of Harissa & tahini hummus (see page 102) with pitta strips
FRIDAY	One Banana muffin (see page 29); 150 ml (¼ pint) glass orange juice	Canned sardines on wholegrain toast; handful of cherry tomatoes	Turkey balls with minty quinoa (see page 141)	Handful of olives; feta cheese cubes
SATURDAY	Granola with peaches and yogurt (see page 21)	Mediterranean-style tomato soup (see page 162); wholegrain toast	Spinach & fish pie (see page 154)	A pear; a few squares of dark chocolate
SUNDAY	Smashed avocado on wholegrain toast, topped with a poached egg	Fig, bean & toasted pecan salad (see page 77)	Baked cod steak served with Baby vegetables with pesto (see page 182)	Handful of walnuts; 2 clementines

Week two

	BREAKFAST	LUNCH	DINNER	SNACKS
MONDAY	Pesto scrambled eggs (see page 32); 150 ml (¼ pint) glass orange juice	Wholegrain wrap filled with cold shredded roast chicken, tomatoes and guacamole	Vegetable spaghetti Bolognese (see page 137)	Couple of Herb oatcakes (see page 96), spread with reduced fat cream cheese; handful of cherry tomatoes
TUESDAY	One Banana muffin (see page 29); bowl of mixed berries	Mediterranean rice salad (see page 53)	Lemony prawns & broccoli stir-fry (see page 129)	One apple; a few squares of dark chocolate
WEDNESDAY	Wholegrain sourdough toast topped with reduced-fat cream cheese and smoked salmon; bowl of mixed berries	Baked sweet potato topped with black beans, salsa and Greek yogurt	Turkey balls with minty quinoa (see page 141); Baby green peppers in olive oil (see page 89)	Heaped tablespoon of Aubergine dip with flatbreads (see page 109)
THURSDAY	Homemade muesli (see page 42) with semi-skimmed milk and chopped banana	Bruschetta with tomatoes & ricotta (see page 105)	Grilled boneless chicken thighs served with Sweet potato & garlic mash (see page 180)	A handful of almonds; one peach or nectarine
FRIDAY	Porridge with semi-skimmed milk, topped with frozen mixed berries (thawed) and a heaped teaspoon nut butter and a drizzle of honey	Smoked mackerel crostini (see page 97); bowl of leafy greens	Mediterranean olive chicken (see page 157)	Handful each of olives; feta cheese cubes
SATURDAY	Potato rösti with frazzled eggs (see page 35); 150 ml (¼ pint) glass of orange juice	Spiced chicken & mango salad (see page 83)	Spinach & fish pie (see page 154) with Baby vegetables with pesto (see page 182)	One apple; a few squares of dark chocolate
SUNDAY	Spinach, potato & ricotta frittata (see page 38); one peach or nectarine	Fig, bean & toasted pecan salad (see page 77)	Spiced mackerel fillets (see page 134) with Mediterranean potato salad (see page 66)	Parsnip & beetroot crisps (see page 106) with salsa

Week three

	BREAKFAST	LUNCH	DINNER	SNACKS
MONDAY	Homemade muesli (see page 42) with natural yogurt and a handful of blueberries and strawberries	Minced turkey salad (see page 58) with a slice of wholegrain bread	Roasted salmon & vegetables (see page 125)	Handful of Chilli, lime & coriander dried fruit & nuts (see page 93); one peach or nectarine
TUESDAY	Florentine-style eggs (see page 45); bowl of mixed berries	Niçoise salad (see page 85)	Spinach & fish pie (see page 154)	One pear; a few squares of dark chocolate
WEDNESDAY	Smashed avocado on wholegrain toast, topped with a poached egg	Tuna & jalapeño baked potatoes (see page 177) topped with a large handful of watercress	Spiced tofu, noodles & pak choi (see page 126)	Parsnip & beetroot crisps (see page 106) with salsa
THURSDAY	Smoothie made with half a banana, big handful each of raspberries and blueberries, heaped teaspoon of nut butter and 150 ml (¼ pint) plant-based or dairy milk	Mediterranean-style tomato soup (see page 162); wholegrain bread	Spicy Mediterranean pasta (see page 153)	Heaped tablespoon of Aubergine dip with flatbreads (see page 109)
FRIDAY	Rice & sweetcorn omelette (see page 46); 150 ml (¼ pint) glass of orange juice	Canned sardines on wholegrain toast with sliced cucumber & carrot	Chargrilled chicken with salsa & fruity couscous (see page 128)	Apple slices with a level tablespoon of nut butter
SATURDAY	Pesto scrambled eggs (see page 32); 150 ml (¼ pint) glass of orange juice	Honeyed pumpkin and ginger broth (see page 173) with toasted wholegrain pitta	Garlic & tomato seafood spaghetti (see page 145)	Heaped tablespoon Greek yogurt with a handful of berries and a teaspoon of chopped mixed nuts
SUNDAY	Granola with peaches and yogurt (see page 21)	Panzanella-style salad (see page 78)	Aubergine bake (see page 150)	Heaped tablespoon Harissa & tahini hummus (see page 102) served with carrot and cucumber sticks

Week four

	BREAKFAST	LUNCH	DINNER	SNACKS
MONDAY	Herby smoked salmon omelettes (see page 22); 150 ml (¼ pint) glass orange juice	Smoked salmon & potato salad (see page 57); bowl of leafy greens; one slice of wholegrain bread	Grilled boneless chicken thighs served with Sweet potato & garlic mash (see page 180)	Small slice of Tropical fruit cake (see page 194); one apple
TUESDAY	Turkey croque madame (see page 26); bowl of mixed berries	Chicken, apricot & almond salad (see page 61)	Mediterranean olive chicken (see page 157)	Heaped tablespoon Greek yogurt with a handful of berries and a teaspoon of chopped mixed nuts
WEDNESDAY	Omelette with basil tomatoes (see page 31)	Wholegrain wrap with cold shredded roast chicken, avocado, lettuce and hummus	Spinach & fish pie (see page 154)	Couple of Herb oatcakes (see page 96), spread with reduced fat cream cheese; handful of cherry tomatoes
THURSDAY	Florentine-style eggs (see page 45)	Spiced tuna open sandwiches served with watercress (see page 170)	Spicy Mediterranean pasta (see page 153)	One apple; a few squares of dark chocolate
FRIDAY	Shredded wheat, served with semi-skimmed milk, chopped banana and chopped nuts	Ciabatta toasties with Mediterranean vegetables (see page 174)	Crusted salmon with tomato salsa (see page 149)	Handful of olives; a few mini mozzarella balls
SATURDAY	Mediterranean-style beans (see page 39)	Fig, bean & toasted pecan salad (see page 77)	Vegetable spaghetti Bolognese (see page 137)	Handful of Chilli, lime & coriander dried fruit & nuts (see page 93); a pear
SUNDAY	Potato rösti with frazzled eggs (see page 35); 150 ml (¼ pint) glass of orange juice	Mushroom risotto cakes (see page 168) served with Carrot & cashew nut salad (see page 65)	Turkey balls with minty quinoa (see page 141)	Heaped tablespoon Harissa & tahini hummus (see page 102) served with carrot and cucumber sticks

Breakfast

21	**granola with peaches & yogurt**
22	**herby smoked salmon omelettes**
23	**poached eggs & spinach**
24	**home-baked seeded rolls**
26	**turkey croque madame**
29	**banana muffins**
31	**omelette with basil tomatoes**
32	**pesto scrambled eggs**
35	**potato rösti with frazzled eggs**
36	**fruit granola bars**
38	**spinach, potato & ricotta frittata**
39	**Mediterranean-style beans**
41	**spinach, tomato & parmesan scones**
42	**homemade muesli**
45	**Florentine-style eggs**
46	**rice & sweetcorn omelette**

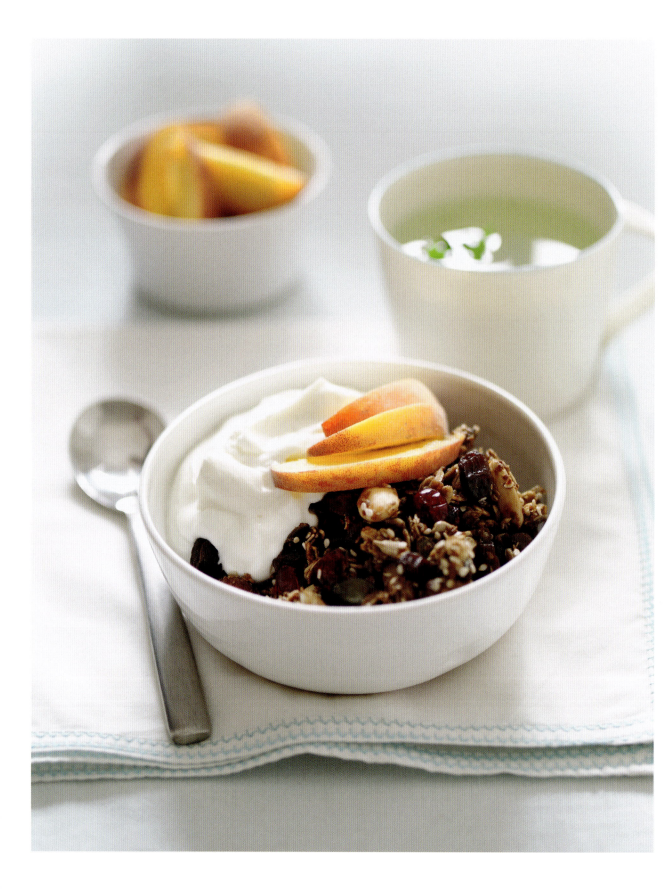

SERVES 4

PREPARATION TIME 15 MINUTES, PLUS COOLING

COOKING TIME 45 MINUTES

Start the day with this nut- and seed-rich granola for a healthy dose of unsaturated fats, antioxidants and fatigue-fighting iron and magnesium.

granola with peaches & yogurt

200 g (7 oz) rolled oats

50 g (2 oz) wheatgerm

50 g (2 oz) sunflower seeds

25 g (1 oz) sesame seeds or linseeds

50 g (2 oz) pumpkin seeds

50 g (2 oz) whole blanched almonds

50 g (2 oz) hazelnuts

½ teaspoon ground cinnamon

½ teaspoon ground mixed spice

¼ teaspoon salt

3 tablespoons maple syrup

1 tablespoon molasses or treacle

2 tablespoons rapeseed oil

75 g (3 oz) ready-to-eat dried apricots, chopped

50 g (2 oz) dried cranberries

50 g (2 oz) sultanas

350 ml (12 fl oz) fat-free Greek yogurt

2 peaches, stoned and sliced

Mix together the cereals, seeds, nuts, spices and salt in a large bowl.

Heat the maple syrup, molasses or treacle, oil and 2 tablespoons water in a small saucepan, then pour over the dry ingredients. Stir until thoroughly combined.

Tip the mixture on to a large, lightly oiled baking sheet, then press down firmly to make clumps. Place in a preheated oven, 140°C (275°F), Gas Mark 1, for about 30 minutes. Add the dried fruits and stir gently to combine. Return to the oven for a further 15 minutes or until evenly crisp and golden brown.

Leave to cool on the baking sheet (it will continue to crisp up as it cools), then store in an airtight container for up to 1 week. To serve, spoon into serving bowls and top with the yogurt and peaches.

SERVES 4

PREPARATION TIME 10 MINUTES

COOKING TIME ABOUT 15 MINUTES

> Combining omega-3 rich salmon with protein-packed eggs makes an anti-inflammatory breakfast that is also very filling.

herby smoked salmon omelettes

8 large eggs

2 spring onions, thinly sliced

2 tablespoons chopped chives

2 tablespoons chopped chervil

50 g (2 oz) butter

4 thin slices of smoked salmon, cut into thin strips, or 125 g (4 oz) smoked salmon trimmings

pepper

baby leaf and herb salad, to serve

Put the eggs, spring onions and herbs in a bowl, beat together lightly and season with pepper.

Heat a medium-sized frying pan over a medium-low heat, add a quarter of the butter and melt until beginning to froth. Pour in a quarter of the egg mixture and swirl to cover the base of the pan. Stir gently for 2–3 minutes or until almost set.

Sprinkle over a quarter of the smoked salmon strips and cook for a further 30 seconds or until just set. Fold over and slide on to a serving plate. Repeat to make 3 more omelettes. Serve each omelette immediately with a baby leaf and herb salad.

FOR SMOKED HAM & TOMATO OMELETTE

Make as above, adding 8–12 quartered cherry tomatoes to the egg mixture. Replace the smoked salmon with 4 thin slices of smoked ham, cut into strips.

SERVES 4
PREPARATION TIME 5 MINUTES
COOKING TIME 8–10 MINUTES

Having some colourful veg on your plate is a great way to start your day. This breakfast counts as one of your five-a-day.

poached eggs & spinach

4 strips of cherry tomatoes on the vine, about 6 tomatoes on each

2 tablespoons balsamic syrup or glaze

1 small bunch of basil, leaves removed

1 tablespoon distilled vinegar

4 large eggs

4 thick slices of wholemeal bread

butter or olive spread (optional)

100 g (3½ oz) baby leaf spinach

salt and pepper

Lay the cherry tomato vines in an ovenproof dish, drizzle with the balsamic syrup or glaze, scatter with the basil leaves and season with salt and pepper. Place in a preheated oven, 180°C (350°F), Gas Mark 4, for 8–10 minutes or until the tomatoes begin to collapse.

Meanwhile, bring a large saucepan of water to a gentle simmer, add the vinegar and stir with a large spoon to create a swirl. Carefully break 2 eggs into the water and cook for 3 minutes. Remove with a slotted spoon and keep warm. Repeat with the remaining eggs.

Toast the wholemeal bread and butter lightly, if liked.

Heap the spinach on to serving plates and top each plate with a poached egg. Arrange the vine tomatoes on the plates, drizzled with any cooking juices. Serve immediately with the wholemeal toast, cut into fingers.

FOR SPINACH, EGG & CRESS SALAD

Gently lower the unshelled eggs into a saucepan of simmering water. Cook for 7–8 minutes, then cool quickly under running cold water. Shell the eggs and slice thickly. Arrange the egg slices over the spinach leaves and halved cherry tomatoes. Scatter with 20 g (¾ oz) salad cress and serve with a little olive oil and balsamic syrup.

MAKES 8 ROLLS

PREPARATION TIME 25 MINUTES, PLUS PROVING

COOKING TIME 12–15 MINUTES

home-baked seeded rolls

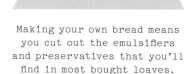

Making your own bread means you cut out the emulsifiers and preservatives that you'll find in most bought loaves.

500 g (1 lb) strong plain or wholegrain bread flour, plus extra for dusting

50 g (2 oz) mixed seeds

1 teaspoon fast-action dried yeast

1 teaspoon sugar

1 teaspoon salt

275 ml (9 fl oz) hand-hot water

1 tablespoon melted butter

oil, for greasing

TO SERVE

thick-cut orange marmalade

freshly squeezed fruit juice (optional)

Put the flour, seeds and yeast in a large bowl, then stir in the sugar and salt. Pour in the measured water and the butter and mix to a dough. Turn the dough out on a lightly floured surface and knead for 5–10 minutes or until smooth and elastic.

Place in a lightly oiled bowl, cover with a clean, slightly damp tea towel and leave in a warm place to rise for at least 1 hour or until doubled in size. Alternatively, make the dough in a bread machine according to the manufacturer's instructions.

Push the dough back down and then divide into 8 balls. Knead each piece until smooth and round, then place evenly spaced on a large, lightly greased baking sheet. Cut a deep cross in each one, cover again with the damp tea towel and leave in a warm place to rise for 1 hour or until doubled in size.

Bake the rolls in a preheated oven, 200°C (400°F), Gas Mark 6, for 12–15 minutes or until golden and crusty and the rolls sound hollow when tapped on the underside. Cool slightly on a wire rack, pulling apart if they have spread during rising or cooking. Serve warm, split in half, with a bowl of thick-cut orange marmalade and a glass of freshly squeezed fruit juice, if liked.

FOR MIXED SEED LOAF

Make the dough as above but form into 1 large, round loaf. Leave to rise until doubled in size and then bake in the oven for 30 minutes or until golden and crusty and the loaf sounds hollow when tapped on the underside. Cool on a wire rack. Cut into slices and serve warm or toasted.

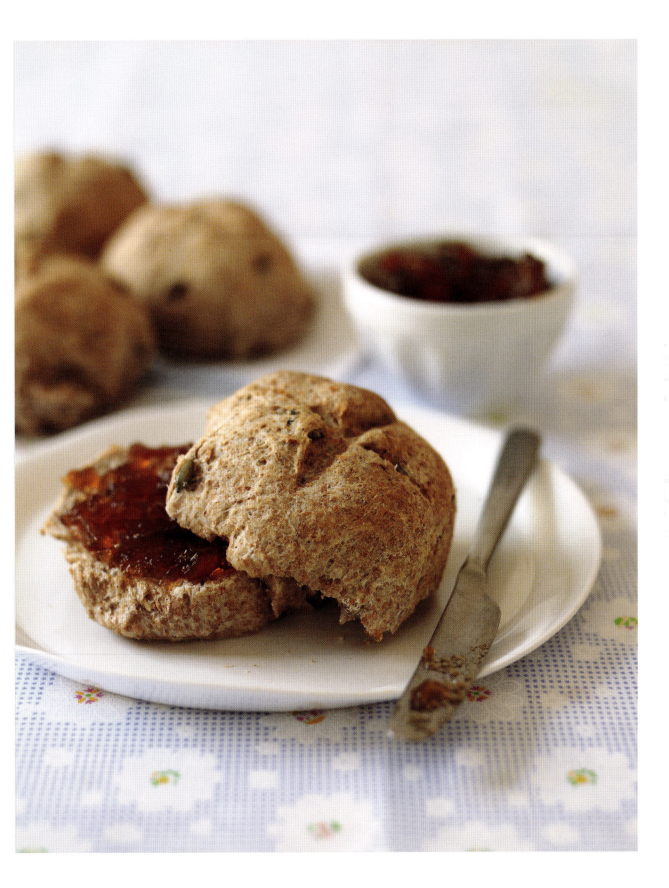

SERVES 4
PREPARATION TIME 10 MINUTES
COOKING TIME 8–10 MINUTES

Though it is best to moderate the amount of cheese in an anti-inflammatory diet, the Cheddar (and spinach) in this recipe provide plenty of calcium, which is important for maintaining strong bones.

turkey croque madame

8 slices of wholegrain bread from a large, round loaf

3 tablespoons wholegrain mustard

200 g (7 oz) aged Gruyère or reduced-fat mature Cheddar cheese, finely grated

200 g (7 oz) cooked turkey, thinly sliced

2 tomatoes, sliced

2 spring onions, thinly sliced

4 tablespoons reduced-fat cream cheese (optional)

1 tablespoon distilled vinegar

4 large eggs

100 g (3½ oz) baby leaf spinach

pepper

chopped chives, to garnish

Spread 4 slices of bread with the mustard. Top with half of the Gruyère or Cheddar, the turkey and tomato slices, then scatter with the spring onions. Season with pepper and scatter over the remaining Gruyère or Cheddar. Spread the cream cheese, if using, over the remaining slices of bread and place, cheese side down, on top of the sandwiches.

Heat a large, nonstick frying pan over a medium heat until hot, then carefully add the sandwiches and cook for 4–5 minutes or until golden and crispy. Turn over and cook for a further 4–5 minutes. Alternatively, toast in a panini machine according to the manufacturer's instructions.

Meanwhile, bring a large saucepan of water to a gentle simmer, add the vinegar and stir with a large spoon to create a swirl. Carefully break 2 eggs into the water and cook for 3 minutes. Remove with a slotted spoon and keep warm. Repeat with the remaining eggs.

Transfer each sandwich to a plate, scatter over a few spinach leaves and top with a poached egg. Garnish with chives and serve immediately.

FOR TURKEY & CHEESE SANDWICHES

Cut 1 large wholegrain baguette almost in half lengthways. Cut into 4 and place, opened out, on a baking sheet. Top as above with the mustard, turkey, tomatoes and spring onions. Omit the cream cheese and finish with all of the grated cheese. Cook under a preheated hot grill for 3–4 minutes or until hot and melted. Serve hot with baby leaf spinach and poached eggs, if liked.

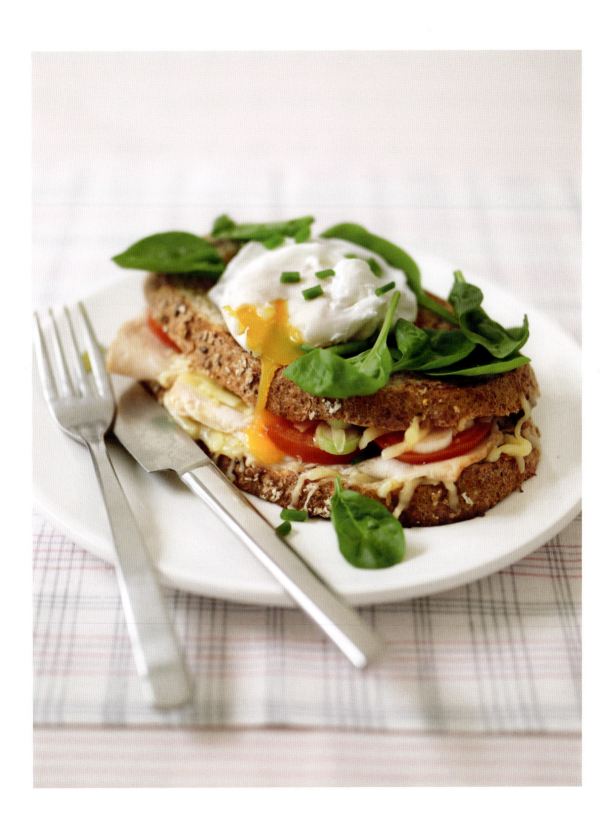

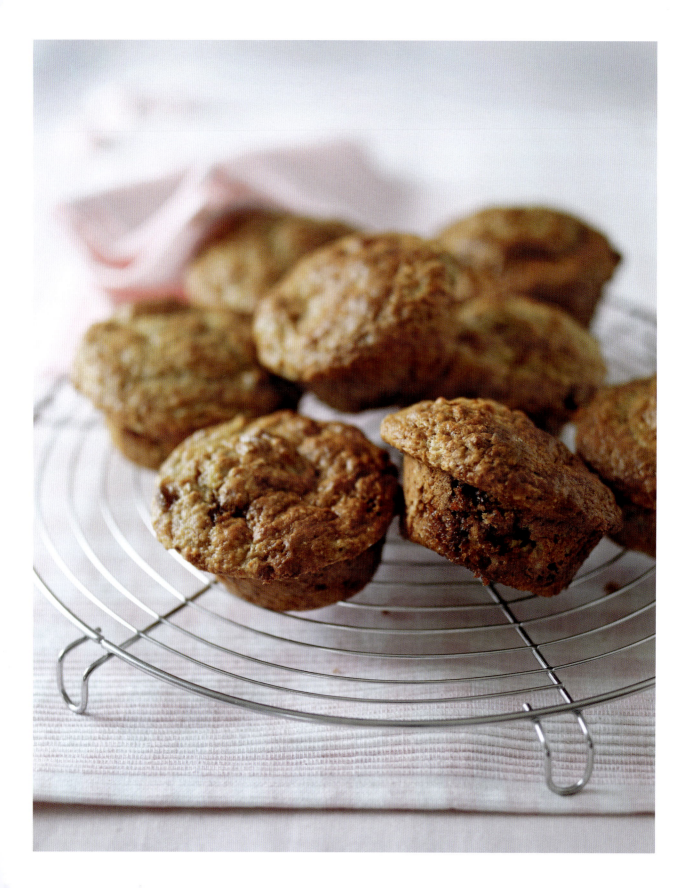

MAKES 12
PREPARATION TIME 10 MINUTES
COOKING TIME 20–22 MINUTES

banana muffins

200 g (7 oz) wholemeal flour

35 g (1½ oz) bran

75 g (3 oz) soft dark brown sugar

1 teaspoon baking powder

¾ teaspoon bicarbonate of soda

½ teaspoon ground mixed spice (optional)

200 ml (7 fl oz) buttermilk

2½ tablespoons groundnut oil

2 large eggs, beaten

1 teaspoon vanilla extract

2 small, very ripe bananas, peeled and mashed

freshly squeezed fruit juice, to serve (optional)

Mix together the dry ingredients in a large bowl. Stir together the remaining ingredients in a separate bowl, then pour the wet ingredients into the dry mixture and stir with a large metal spoon until just combined.

Spoon the mixture into a lightly greased large, 12-hole nonstick muffin tray, or alternatively, a 6-hole tray, and bake in a preheated oven, 180°C (350°F), Gas Mark 4, for 20–22 minutes or until risen and golden and a skewer inserted into the centres comes out clean.

Transfer to a wire rack to cool slightly. Serve the still-warm muffins with glasses of freshly squeezed fruit juice, if liked.

FOR BANANA, BLUEBERRY & WHEATGERM MUFFINS

Make as above, replacing 1 of the bananas with 125 g (4 oz) blueberries, the bran with 35 g (1½ oz) wheatgerm and the mixed spice with ½ teaspoon ground cinnamon.

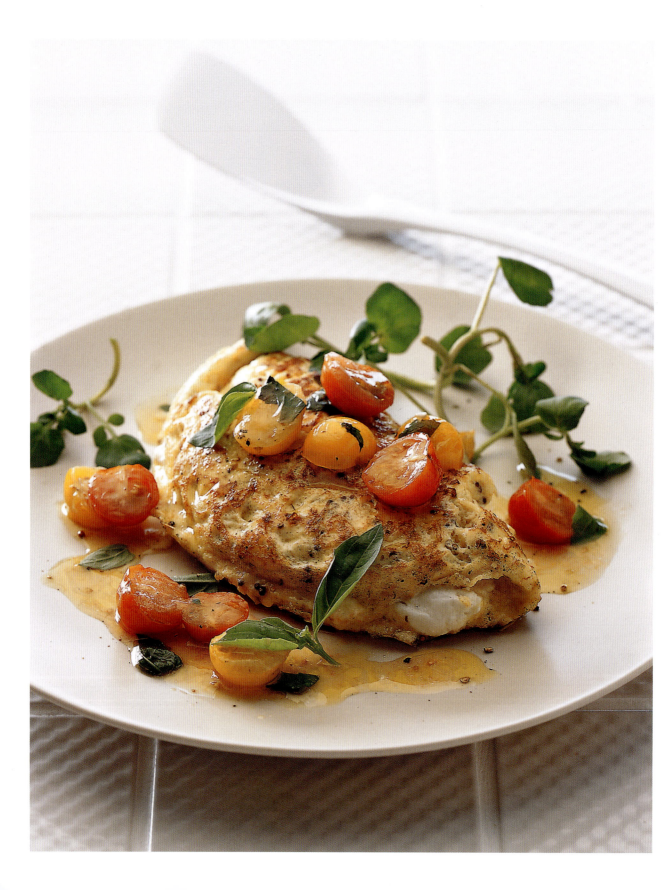

SERVES 4
PREPARATION TIME 10 MINUTES
COOKING TIME 16–20 MINUTES

omelette with basil tomatoes

4 tablespoons extra virgin olive oil

500 g (1 lb) cherry tomatoes, halved

a few chopped basil leaves

12 eggs

2 tablespoons wholegrain mustard

50 g (2 oz) butter

100 g (3½ oz) soft goats' cheese, diced

salt and pepper

watercress, to garnish

green salad, to serve

Heat the oil in a large frying pan, add the tomatoes, in batches if necessary, and cook, stirring gently, for 2–3 minutes until softened. Add the basil and season with salt and pepper. Transfer to a bowl and keep warm in a moderate oven.

Beat the eggs, mustard and salt and pepper together in a separate bowl. Melt a quarter of the butter in an omelette pan or small frying pan. As soon as it stops foaming, swirl in a quarter of the egg mixture and cook over a medium heat, forking over the omelette so that it cooks evenly.

Dot a quarter of the goats' cheese over one half of the omelette as soon as it is set on the underside, but still a little runny in the centre, and cook for a further 30 seconds. Carefully slide the omelette on to a warmed serving plate, folding it in half as you go. Keep warm in the oven. Repeat with the remaining egg mixture to make 3 more omelettes.

Garnish the omelettes with watercress and serve with the tomatoes and a green salad.

FOR TOMATO-STUFFED OMELETTE

Omit the first step of the above recipe. Arrange a quarter of the tomatoes with the goats' cheese over one half of the omelette as soon as it is set on the underside. Follow the recipe above to finish the omelette and then serve with a rocket salad.

SERVES 4
PREPARATION TIME 5 MINUTES
COOKING TIME 5 MINUTES

> Basil pesto amps up the anti-inflammatory nature of this dish. Making your own pesto with a big pile of fresh basil (see below) is the healthiest option.

pesto scrambled eggs

12 eggs

100 ml (3½ fl oz) single cream

25 g (1 oz) butter

4 slices of granary bread, toasted

4 tablespoons Pesto (see below)

salt and pepper

Beat the eggs, cream and a little salt and pepper together in a bowl. Melt the butter in a large, nonstick frying pan, add the egg mixture and stir over a low heat with a wooden spoon until cooked to your liking.

Put a slice of toast on each serving plate. Spoon a quarter of the scrambled eggs on to each slice of toast, make a small indent in the centre and add a tablespoonful of pesto. Serve immediately.

FOR HOMEMADE PESTO

Put 50 g (2 oz) basil leaves, 1 garlic clove, 4 tablespoons pine nuts, 100 ml (3½ fl oz) extra virgin oil and salt and pepper in a food processor and process until fairly smooth. Transfer to a bowl, stir in 2 tablespoons freshly grated Parmesan cheese and adjust the seasoning.

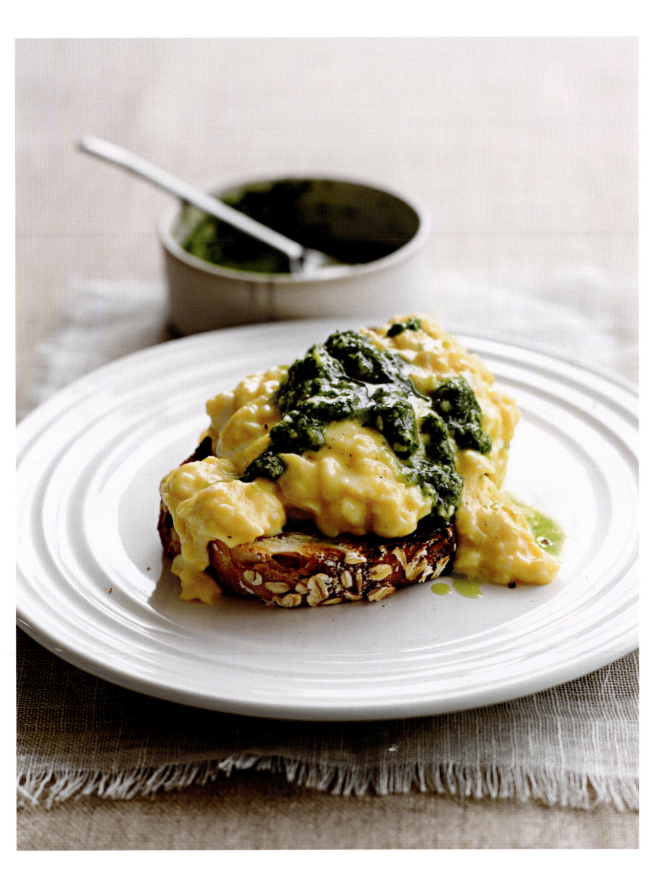

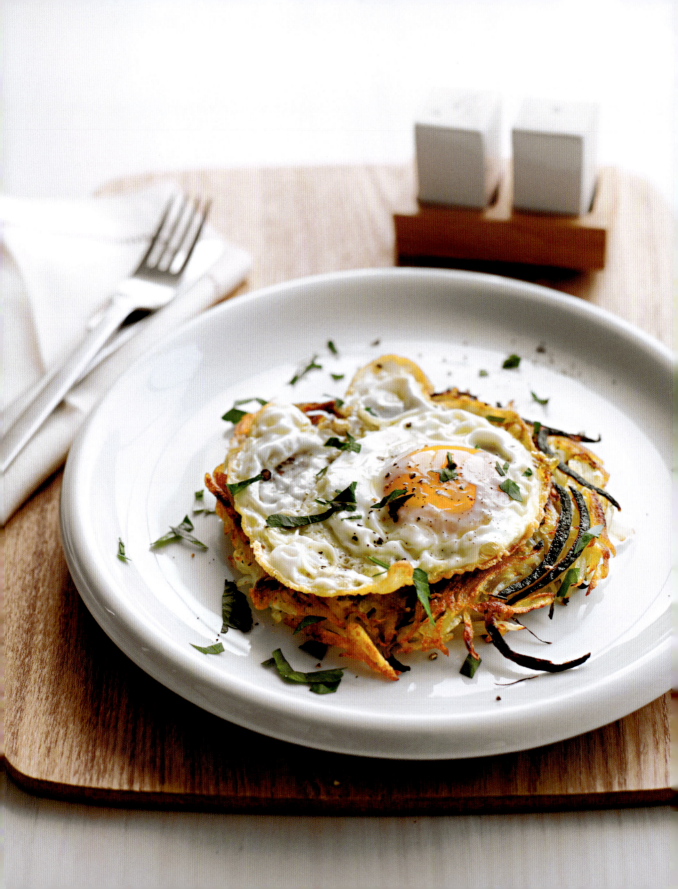

SERVES 4

PREPARATION TIME 15 MINUTES

COOKING TIME 15 MINUTES

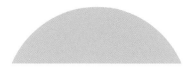

Eggs contain vitamin D — the sunshine vitamin — which helps with your bone, muscle and gut microbiome health.

potato rösti with frazzled eggs

750 g (1½ lb) Désirée potatoes, peeled

1 onion, thinly sliced

2 teaspoons chopped rosemary

4 tablespoons olive oil

4 large eggs

salt and pepper

chopped parsley, to garnish

Using a box grater, coarsely grate the potatoes. Wrap in a clean tea towel and squeeze out the excess liquid over the sink. Transfer to a bowl and stir in the onion, rosemary and salt and pepper.

Heat half the oil in a large frying pan. Divide the potato mixture into quarters and spoon into 4 x 12 cm (5 inch) mounds in the pan, pressing down to form patties. Cook the patties over a medium heat for 5 minutes on each side, transfer to warmed serving plates and keep warm in a moderate oven.

Heat the remaining oil in the frying pan for about 1 minute until very hot, add the eggs, 2 at a time, and fry until the whites are bubbly and crisp looking. Serve the eggs on the rösti, garnished with chopped parsley.

FOR RÖSTI WITH POACHED EGGS

Bring a saucepan of lightly salted water to a simmer and add 1 tablespoon white vinegar. Crack an egg into a cup. Swirl the simmering water with a large spoon, gently drop the egg into the centre and cook for 2–3 minutes. Carefully remove with a slotted spoon. Repeat with the remaining eggs and finish as above.

MAKES 9

PREPARATION TIME 20 MINUTES, PLUS COOLING

COOKING TIME 40 MINUTES

fruit granola bars

225 g (7½ oz) peeled, cored and roughly chopped dessert apple

1 tablespoon lemon juice

½ teaspoon ground cinnamon

sunflower oil, for oiling

GRANOLA

125 g (4 oz) rolled oats

125 g (4 oz) ready-to-eat dried apricots

125 g (4 oz) fresh Medjool dates, stoned and roughly chopped

2 tablespoons ground flaxseed (linseed)

2 tablespoons smooth peanut butter

2 tablespoons agave syrup

Line a baking sheet with baking parchment. Toss the apple with the lemon juice, agave syrup and cinnamon in a bowl, then spread out on the lined baking sheet and roast in a preheated oven, 160°C (325°F), Gas Mark 3, for 20 minutes. Remove from the oven and leave to cool.

Increase the oven temperature to 180°C (350°F), Gas Mark 4. Pulse all the ingredients for the granola together in a food processor a few times until mixed and mashed. Fold in the cooled roasted apple, then spoon into a lightly oiled 20 cm (8 inch) square shallow cake tin and level with the back of a spoon. Bake in the oven for 20 minutes.

Leave to cool for 15 minutes before cutting into 9 squares to serve.

FOR PEAR, BANANA & HAZELNUT GRANOLA BARS

Toss 225 g (7½ oz) peeled, cored and chopped pear with 1 tablespoon each lemon juice and agave syrup in a bowl, then spread out on a baking sheet lined with baking parchment and roast in a preheated oven, 180°C (350°F), Gas Mark 4 for 20 minutes. Remove from the oven and leave to cool, keeping the oven on. Pulse together 125 g (4 oz) each rolled oats and fresh Medjool dates, stoned and roughly chopped, 1 small ripe banana, roughly chopped, 2 tablespoons each ground flaxseed (linseed) and toasted blanched hazelnuts and 55 ml (2 fl oz) agave syrup in a food processor a few times until mixed and mashed. Fold in the cooled roasted pear, then bake, cool and cut into squares as above.

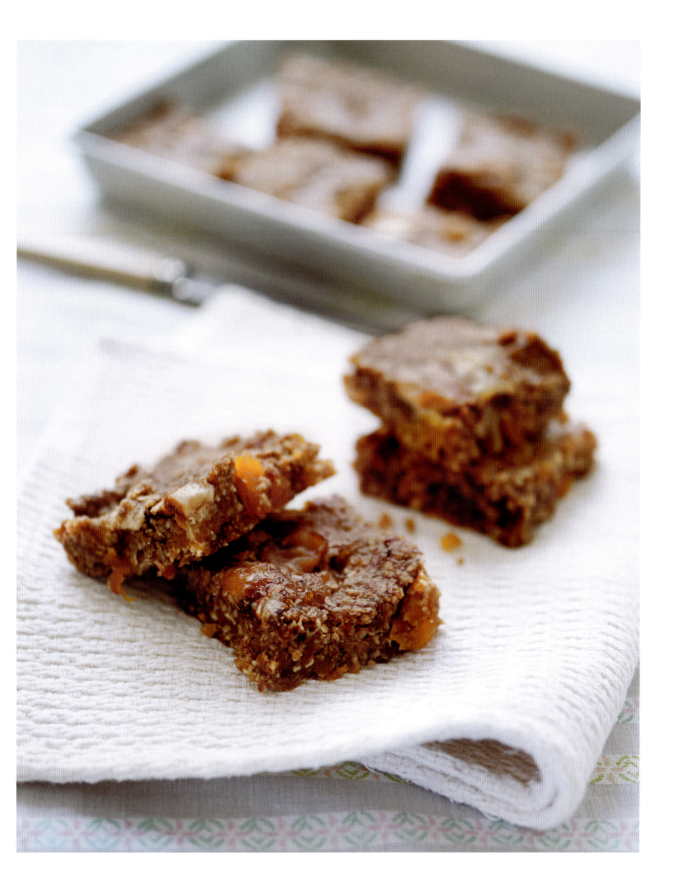

SERVES 4
PREPARATION TIME 1 MINUTE
COOKING TIME 7–9 MINUTES

Don't have any fresh spinach? Frozen works just as well and is equally as nutritious.

spinach, potato & ricotta frittata

200 g (7 oz) new potatoes, scrubbed and thinly sliced

1 tablespoon olive oil

100 g (3½ oz) baby spinach

6 eggs

2 tablespoons snipped chives

125 g (4 oz) ricotta cheese

salt and pepper

Cook the potatoes in a saucepan of lightly salted boiling water for 2–3 minutes until just tender. Meanwhile, heat the oil in a 28 cm (11 inch) ovenproof frying pan, add the spinach and cook for 1 minute until wilted.

Beat the eggs in a small bowl with the chives and season to taste. Drain the potatoes and stir into the pan with the spinach, then add the eggs and stir briefly. Cook without stirring over a medium heat for 3–4 minutes until almost set.

Dot the ricotta over the frittata and continue to cook under a preheated hot grill for 2 minutes until golden. Cut into wedges and serve immediately.

FOR SWEETCORN & ROASTED PEPPER FRITTATA

Heat 1 tablespoon olive oil in a frying pan as above, then stir in 150 g (5 oz) chopped ready-roasted red peppers and 200 g (7 oz) canned sweetcorn and cook for 1 minute. Beat 6 eggs with 2 tablespoons chopped parsley and season to taste. Pour into the pan and cook as above, then sprinkle with 125 g (4 oz) grated Cheddar cheese and grill until golden.

SERVES 4
PREPARATION TIME 10 MINUTES
COOKING TIME 10 MINUTES

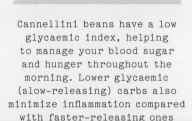

Cannellini beans have a low glycaemic index, helping to manage your blood sugar and hunger throughout the morning. Lower glycaemic (slow-releasing) carbs also minimize inflammation compared with faster-releasing ones that create it.

Mediterranean-style beans

2 tablespoons extra virgin olive oil

1 red onion, diced

1 garlic clove, crushed

½ teaspoon cumin seeds

400 g (13 oz) can cannellini beans, rinsed and drained

75 g (3 oz) cherry tomatoes, quartered

2 teaspoons chopped sage

4 slices of crusty bread

salt and pepper

25 g (1 oz) Manchego cheese, grated, to serve

Heat the oil in a large frying pan, add the red onion and cook for 1–2 minutes. Add the garlic and cumin seeds and cook for a further 2–3 minutes.

Add the beans and mix well to allow them to soak up the flavours, then add the tomatoes. Stir in the sage, season with salt and pepper and heat through.

Meanwhile, toast the bread under a preheated hot grill for 2–3 minutes on each side. Serve topped with the beans and a sprinkling of cheese.

FOR MIXED BEAN GOULASH

Heat 1 tablespoon olive oil in a large frying pan, add 1 large chopped onion and 2 crushed garlic cloves and gently fry for 5 minutes until softened. Stir in 100 g (3½ oz) chopped chestnut mushrooms and cook for a further 3–4 minutes. Add 1 tablespoon smoked paprika and continue to cook for 1–2 minutes. Stir in a 400 g (13 oz) can chopped tomatoes, 200 ml (7 fl oz) hot vegetable stock and a 400 g (13 oz) can mixed beans, rinsed and drained. Bring to the boil, then reduce the heat and simmer for 12–14 minutes until thick and glossy. Serve with cooked rice, topped with dollops of soured cream, if liked.

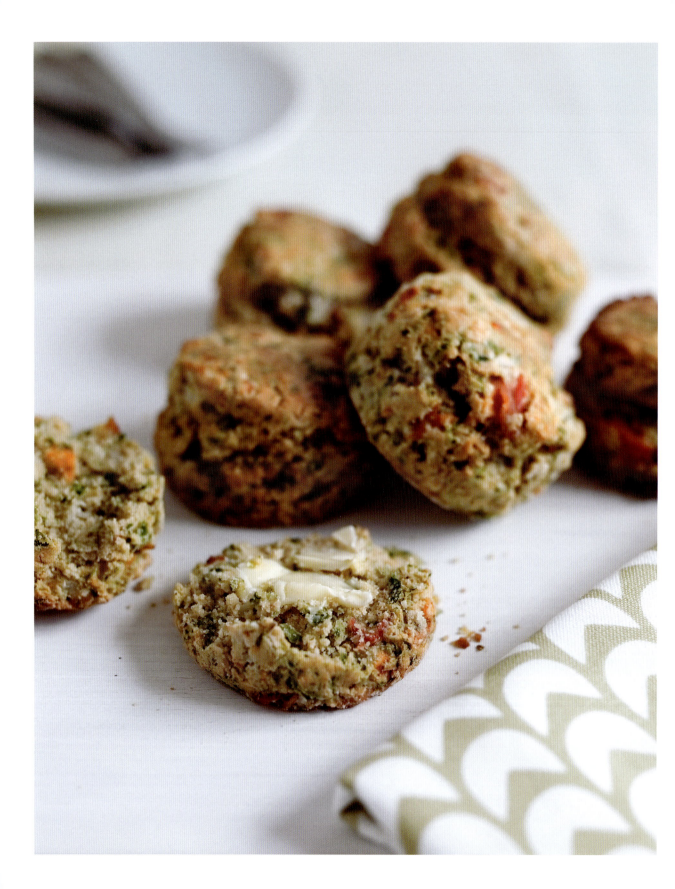

MAKES 8
PREPARATION TIME 10 MINUTES
COOKING TIME 12–15 MINUTES

spinach, tomato & parmesan scones

175 g (6 oz) wholemeal flour, plus extra for dusting

75 g (3 oz) cornflour

1 teaspoon baking powder

1 teaspoon bicarbonate of soda

75 g (3 oz) butter, cubed, plus extra (optional) to serve

100 g (3½ oz) frozen leaf spinach, thawed, squeezed of any liquid and chopped

4 sun-dried tomatoes in oil, drained and finely chopped

50 g (2 oz) Parmesan cheese, grated

good grating of nutmeg

1 large egg, beaten

3 tablespoons buttermilk, plus extra for brushing

Place the flour, cornflour, baking powder, bicarbonate of soda and butter in a food processor and whizz until the mixture resembles fine breadcrumbs. Alternatively, mix together the dry ingredients in a large bowl. Add the butter and rub in with the fingertips until the mixture resembles fine breadcrumbs. Mix in the spinach, sun-dried tomatoes, Parmesan and nutmeg.

Whisk together the egg and buttermilk with a fork in a separate bowl, stir in the flour mixture and combine to form a soft dough.

Turn the dough out on a surface lightly dusted with flour, press out to a thickness of 2.5 cm (1 inch) and use a 5 cm (2 inch) cutter to stamp out 8 scones, re-rolling the trimmings as necessary.

Put on a baking sheet lightly dusted with flour, brush with a little buttermilk and place in a preheated oven, 220°C (425°F), Gas Mark 7, for 12–15 minutes until risen and golden. Serve warm, spread with butter or to accompany a soup.

FOR OLIVE, FETA & HERB SCONES

Make the dough as above, omitting the spinach, sun-dried tomatoes and nutmeg and replacing with 18 sliced pitted olives, 100 g (3½ oz) crumbled feta cheese and 1 tablespoon chopped fresh herbs. Continue as above.

SERVES 4
PREPARATION TIME 5 MINUTES
COOKING TIME 20 MINUTES, PLUS COOLING

> This no-added-sugar muesli is high in all the anti-inflammatory good stuff — fibre, plant proteins and antioxidants.

homemade muesli

100 g (3½ oz) desiccated coconut

250 g (8 oz) buckwheat flakes

250 g (8 oz) millet flakes

100 g (3½ oz) flaked almonds

100 g (3½ oz) blanched hazelnuts

100 g (3½ oz) sunflower seeds

100 g (3½ oz) dried mango, sliced

100 g (3½ oz) sultanas

Spread the coconut out in a thin layer on a baking sheet. Toast in a preheated oven, 150°C (300°F), Gas Mark 2, for about 20 minutes, stirring every 5 minutes to make sure it browns evenly. Toast the flaked almonds, hazelnuts and sunflower seeds in the same way, but be careful not to allow the seeds to burn. Leave to cool, then roughly chop the hazelnuts.

Mix together all the ingredients in a large bowl until well combined. Store in an airtight container for up to 1–2 weeks.

FOR BIRCHER MUESLI

Mix together the millet flakes, dried mango and sultanas with 1 cored and grated red apple in a large bowl. Pour over 300 ml (½ pint) apple juice, cover and chill overnight. Stir in 200 g (7 oz) toasted and roughly chopped mixed nuts, 125 ml (4 fl oz) natural yogurt and a good drizzle of runny honey before serving.

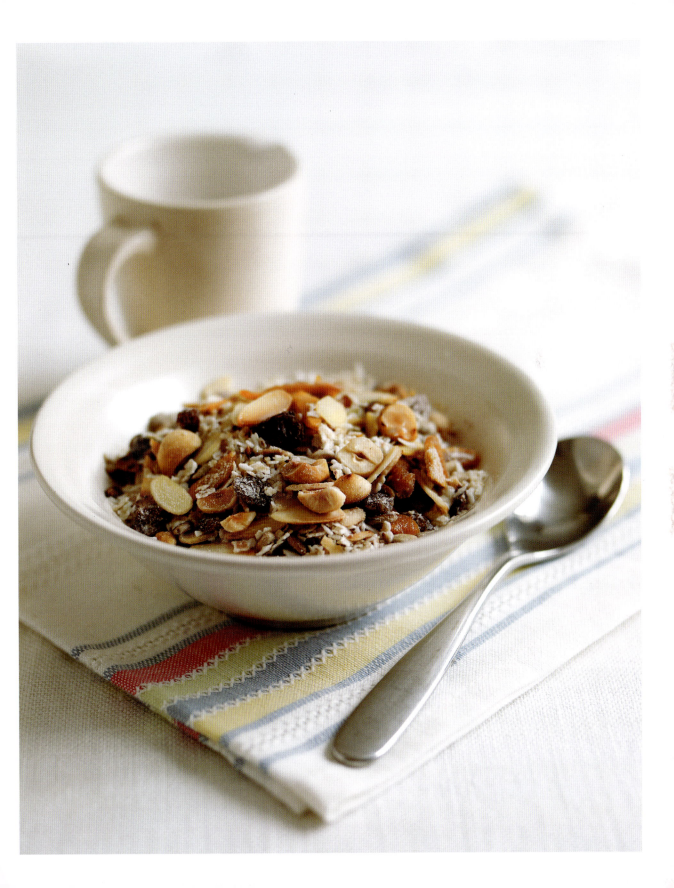

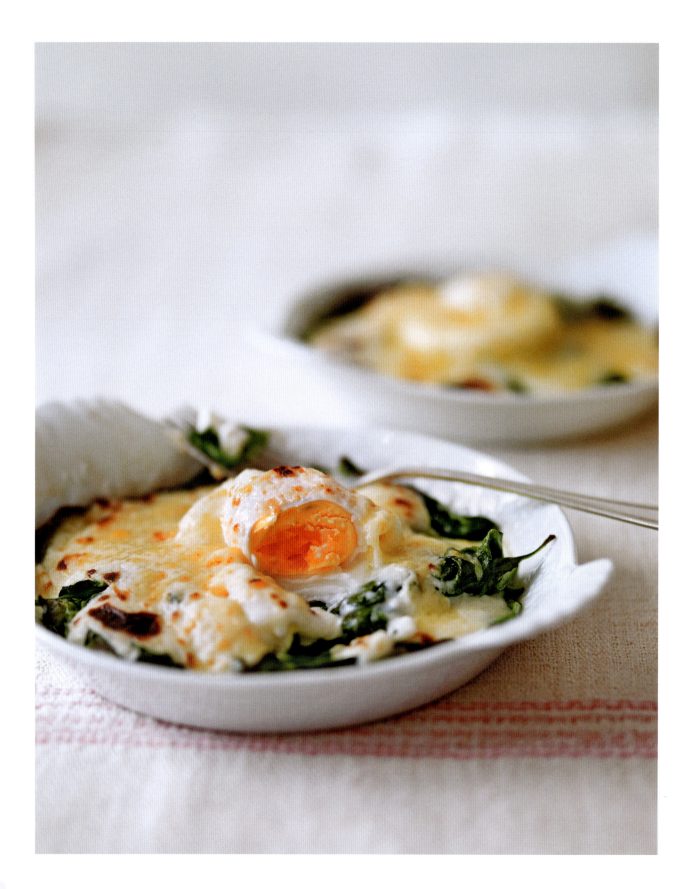

SERVES 4

PREPARATION TIME 5 MINUTES

COOKING TIME 5–10 MINUTES

Florentine-style eggs

450 g (14½ oz) spinach leaves

15 g (½ oz) butter, melted

pinch of grated nutmeg

4 large eggs

salt and pepper

FOR THE CHEESE SAUCE

20 g (¾ oz) butter

20 g (¾ oz) plain flour

¼ teaspoon English mustard

300 ml (½ pint) milk

75 g (3 oz) strong Cheddar cheese, grated

To make the cheese sauce, melt the butter in a small saucepan then stir in the flour and mustard. Cook, stirring continuously, for 1 minute.

Pour in the milk gradually, whisking to remove any lumps, then cook over a gentle heat, stirring continuously, until it begins to boil. Turn the heat down to a simmer and stir in two-thirds of the Cheddar.

Meanwhile, put the spinach in a saucepan with the melted butter and cook for a few minutes. Season with salt and pepper, then add the nutmeg. Place in an ovenproof dish, or divide between 4 individual ovenproof dishes.

Poach the eggs in a frying pan of simmering water for 4–5 minutes, then drain and place them on top of the spinach.

Pour over the cheese sauce and sprinkle with the remaining Cheddar. Place under a preheated hot grill and cook until golden and bubbling. Serve immediately.

SERVES 4
PREPARATION TIME 5 MINUTES
COOKING TIME 10 MINUTES

rice & sweetcorn omelette

15 g (½ oz) butter

4 spring onions, shredded

1 red chilli, deseeded and finely sliced (optional)

200 g (7 oz) can sweetcorn, drained

200 g (7 oz) cooked brown basmati rice

handful of fresh herbs, chopped

6 eggs, beaten

3 tablespoons grated Parmesan cheese

salt and pepper

Heat the butter in a large frying pan, add the spring onions and chilli, if using, and fry for 2 minutes. Add the sweetcorn, rice and herbs and stir to combine.

Pour in the eggs, season well and cook for 2–3 minutes until beginning to set.

Sprinkle over the Parmesan, then place under a preheated hot grill and cook until firm and golden.

Turn out and cut into generous wedges to serve.

FOR CHORIZO & POTATO OMELETTE

Heat 1 tablespoon olive oil in a frying pan, add 1 sliced onion and fry for 3–4 minutes until softened. Add 125 g (4 oz) chopped chorizo sausage and fry for a further 2 minutes until it begins to crisp. Stir in 300 g (10 oz) cooked sliced potatoes and a handful of chopped parsley. Stir to combine, then pour in the beaten eggs. Cook under a hot grill as above.

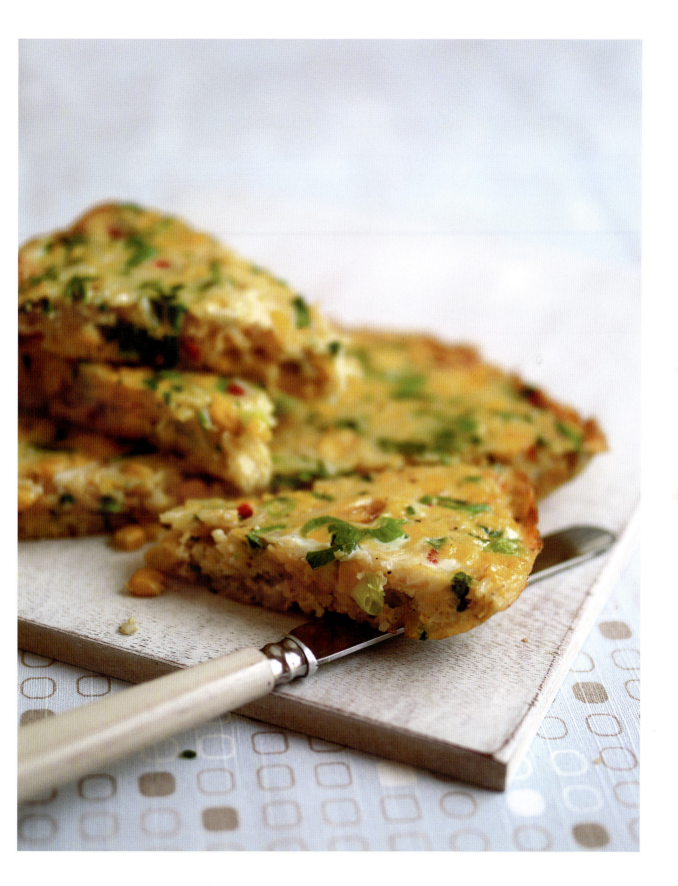

Salads & Leafy Greens

50	**pumpkin, feta & pine nut salad**
53	**Mediterranean rice salad**
54	**cannellini & green bean salad**
57	**smoked salmon & potato salad**
58	**minced turkey salad**
59	**pickled vegetable salad**
61	**chicken, apricot & almond salad**
62	**watermelon, feta & herb salad**
65	**carrot & cashew nut salad**
66	**Mediterranean potato salad**
69	**chickpea & feta salad**
70	**warm lentil, tomato & onion salad**
73	**gingered tofu & mango salad**
74	**Greek-style salad**
77	**fig, bean & toasted pecan salad**
78	**panzanella-style salad**
81	**beetroot & orange salad**
82	**chicken couscous salad**
83	**spiced chicken & mango salad**
85	**Niçoise salad**

SERVES 4

PREPARATION TIME 20 MINUTES

COOKING TIME ABOUT 25 MINUTES

Pine nuts are one of the top plant sources of zinc, which helps protect the genetic material in our cells from oxidation damage.

pumpkin, feta & pine nut salad

500 g (1 lb) pumpkin

olive oil

2 sprigs of thyme, roughly chopped

200 g (7 oz) mixed baby salad leaves

50 g (2 oz) feta cheese

salt and pepper

2 tablespoons toasted pine nuts, to garnish

DRESSING

1 teaspoon Dijon mustard

2 tablespoons balsamic vinegar

4 tablespoons olive oil

Skin and deseed the pumpkin, cut the flesh into 2 cm (¾ inch) squares and put them in a roasting tin. Drizzle with olive oil, scatter over the thyme and season with salt and pepper. Roast the pumpkin in a preheated oven, 190°C (375°F), Gas Mark 5, for 25 minutes or until cooked though. Remove the pumpkin from the oven and allow to cool slightly.

Meanwhile, make the dressing. Whisk together the mustard, vinegar and oil and set aside.

Put the mixed leaves in a large salad bowl, add the cooked pumpkin and crumble in the feta. Drizzle over the dressing and toss carefully to combine. Transfer the mixture to serving plates, garnish with toasted pine nuts and serve immediately.

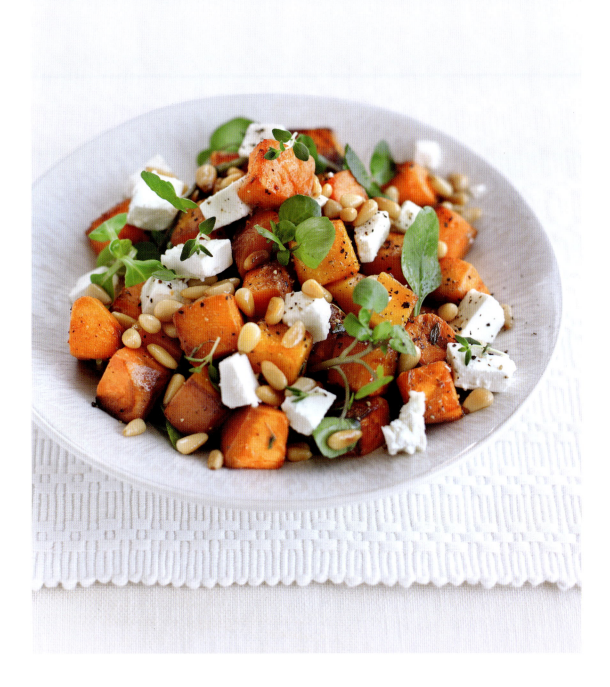

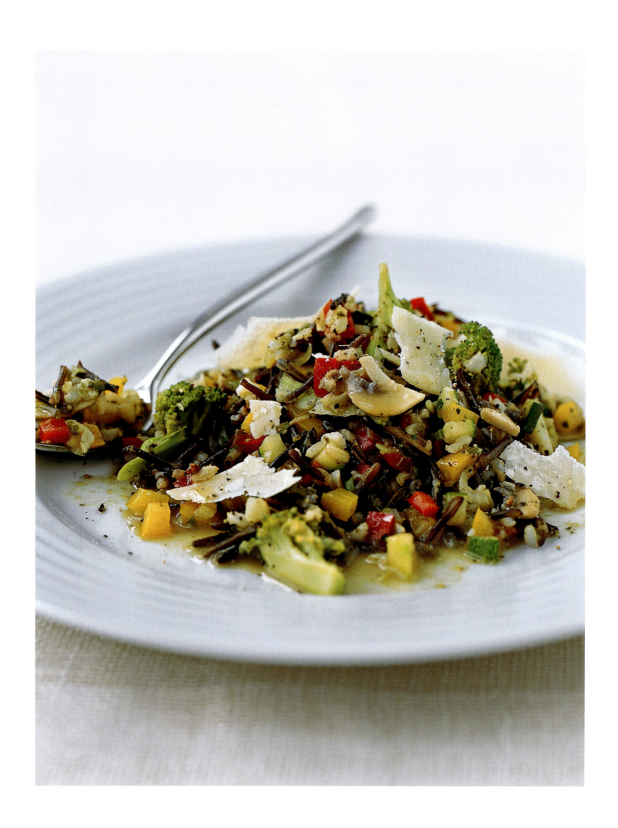

SERVES 4

PREPARATION TIME 10 MINUTES

COOKING TIME 5 MINUTES

Wild and brown rice spike your blood sugar a lot less than white rice, making this salad a good choice for keeping inflammation in check.

Mediterranean rice salad

75 g (3 oz) broccoli, finely chopped

75 g (3 oz) courgettes, finely chopped

75 g (3 oz) mixed red and yellow peppers, finely chopped

25 g (1 oz) spring onions, finely chopped

40 g (1½ oz) mushrooms, finely sliced

2 tablespoons water

2 tablespoons pesto (see page 32)

50 g (2 oz) cooked brown rice

50 g (2 oz) cooked wild rice

salt and pepper

TO SERVE

Parmesan cheese shavings

basil leaves (optional)

Heat a large frying pan or wok, add the vegetables and the measured water and cook over a high heat for 3—5 minutes, until the vegetables have softened. Remove from the heat and allow to cool.

Mix the cooled vegetables with the pesto and cooked rice, season well and stir to combine. Cover and chill until required. Serve topped with a few Parmesan shavings and some basil leaves, if liked.

FOR MEDITERRANEAN PASTA SALAD

Cook the vegetables as above. Meanwhile, cook 150 g (5 oz) macaroni in lightly salted boiling water until just tender. Mix 4 tablespoons olive oil with 1 tablespoon red wine vinegar, 1 finely chopped garlic clove, 2 teaspoons sun-dried tomato paste and a small bunch torn basil leaves. Season well and toss with the pasta and the vegetables.

SERVES 4
PREPARATION TIME 15 MINUTES
COOKING TIME 12–15 MINUTES

Whole (unrefined) carbohydrates like beans and new potatoes help energize you without causing inflammation.

cannellini & green bean salad

300 g (10 oz) small new potatoes, scrubbed and halved

200 g (7 oz) fine green beans, topped and tailed and halved

400 g (13 oz) can cannellini beans, drained and rinsed

75 g (3 oz) pitted black olives, sliced

½ small red onion, thinly sliced

4 tablespoons extra virgin olive oil

grated rind and juice of 1 large lemon

pinch of caster sugar

2 tablespoons chopped mint

2 tablespoons chopped flat leaf parsley

salt and pepper

Cook the potatoes in a large saucepan of boiling water for 12–15 minutes until tender, adding the green beans for the last 3 minutes. Drain and refresh under cold running water.

Place the cannellini beans, olives and onion in a large bowl and stir in the potatoes and green beans.

Whisk together the oil, lemon rind and juice, sugar and salt and pepper in a jug, then stir in the chopped herbs. Pour over the bean and potato mixture and toss well before serving.

FOR WHITE BEAN & TOMATO SALAD

Place 2 x 400 g (13 oz) cans cannellini or butter beans, drained and rinsed, in a bowl and stir in 250 g (8 oz) halved vine cherry tomatoes and 2 tablespoons chopped flat leaf parsley. Whisk together 4 tablespoons extra virgin olive oil, the juice of 1 lemon, 1 teaspoon Dijon mustard and 1 crushed garlic clove in a jug. Season to taste with salt and pepper. Pour over the bean and tomato mixture and gently toss together. Serve with toasted ciabatta, if liked.

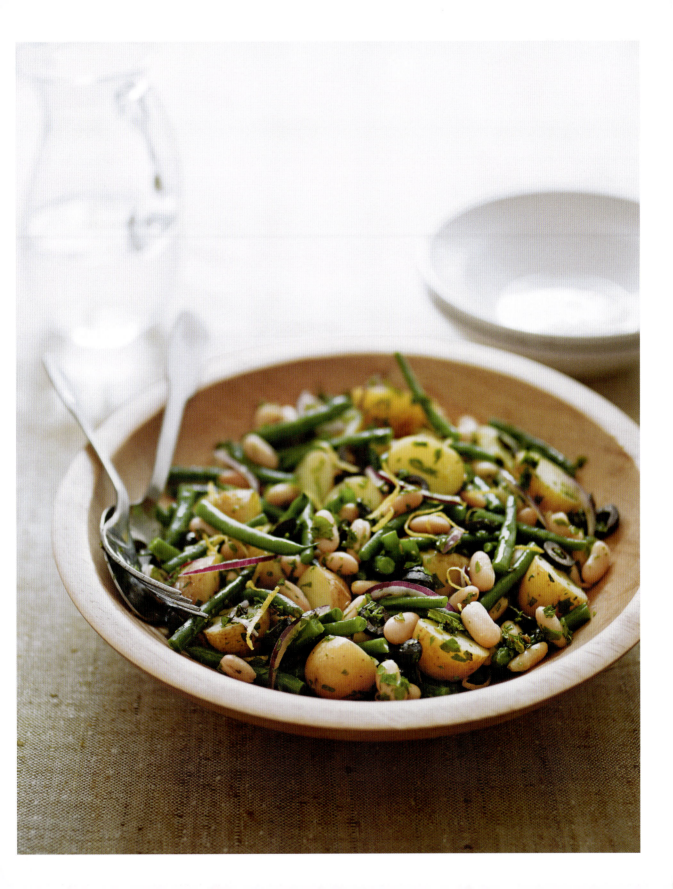

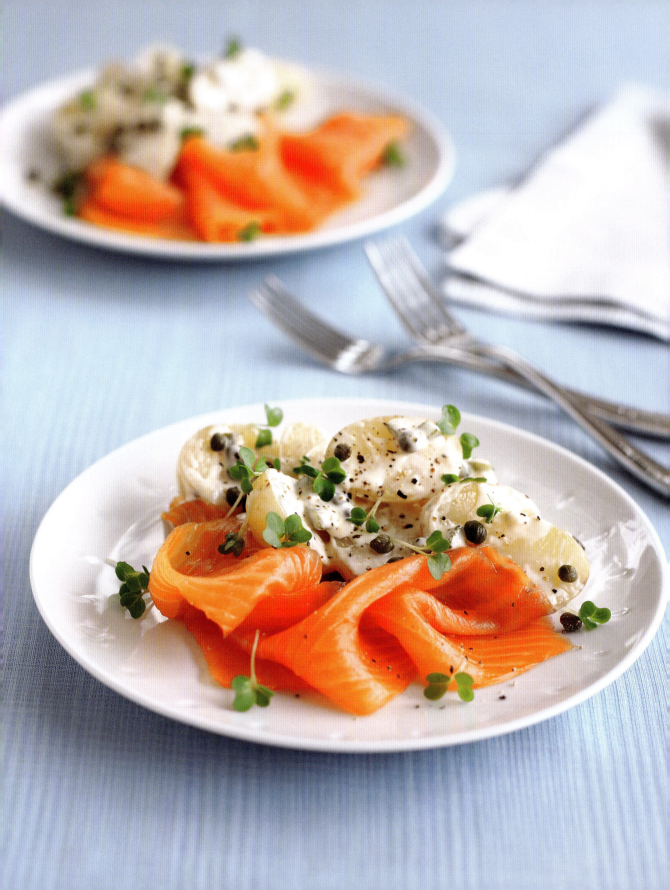

SERVES 4
PREPARATION TIME 15 MINUTES
COOKING TIME 20 MINUTES

smoked salmon & potato salad

600 g (1¼ lb) new potatoes, scrubbed

2 tablespoons small capers

3 tablespoons mayonnaise

2 tablespoons lemon juice

1 teaspoon grated horseradish

150 g (5 oz) smoked salmon

punnet of mustard and cress, trimmed

salt and pepper

Put the potatoes in a saucepan of lightly salted cold water, bring to the boil and cook for 15–20 minutes or until just cooked through. Drain the potatoes and let them cool slightly.

Meanwhile, chop the capers and combine them with the mayonnaise, lemon juice and horseradish. Season to taste with salt and pepper. Put the warm potatoes in a large salad bowl, add the mayonnaise dressing and stir to combine thoroughly.

Arrange the salmon on 4 plates, top with the potatoes and garnish with mustard and cress.

FOR ROAST BEEF & WHOLEGRAIN MUSTARD POTATO SALAD

Seal a 450 g (14½ oz) piece of rib-eye fillet until golden, then cook in a preheated oven, 180°C (350°F), Gas Mark 4, for 15 minutes until cooked to medium rare. Remove, cover with foil and allow to rest. Mix 50 ml (2 fl oz) mayonnaise, 2 tablespoons wholegrain mustard, 1 teaspoon Dijon mustard and 5 finely sliced spring onions. Mix through 600 g (1¼ lb) cooked new potatoes and combine well. Thinly slice the beef and serve with the mustard potato salad.

SERVES 4

PREPARATION TIME 20 MINUTES

COOKING TIME 8–10 MINUTES

minced turkey salad

500 g (1 lb) minced turkey

2 garlic cloves, finely chopped

1 shallot, finely chopped

1 small red chilli, deseeded and finely chopped

1½ tablespoons groundnut oil

½ Chinese cabbage, shredded

150 g (5 oz) mangetout, shredded

½ small cucumber, cut into thin matchsticks

250 g (8 oz) bean sprouts

1 carrot, peeled and cut into thin matchsticks

3 spring onions, thinly sliced

4 tablespoons unsalted peanuts, chopped

chopped fresh coriander

DRESSING

1½ teaspoons peeled and grated fresh root ginger

1½ teaspoons fish sauce

1 tablespoon light soy sauce

2 tablespoons lime juice

2 tablespoons groundnut oil

1½ teaspoons palm sugar

Mix together the turkey, garlic, shallot and chilli in a bowl. Heat the oil in a large frying pan over a medium-high heat, add the turkey mixture and then stir-fry for 8–10 minutes or until the meat is browned and cooked through. Tip into a large bowl.

Whisk together all the dressing ingredients in a small bowl and pour over the cooked turkey. Leave to cool for 10 minutes.

Meanwhile, mix together the Chinese cabbage, mangetout, cucumber, bean sprouts, carrot and spring onions in a bowl. Pile on to serving plates and spoon over the turkey. Sprinkle with the peanuts and coriander and serve immediately.

SERVES 4
PREPARATION TIME 20 MINUTES, PLUS COOLING
COOKING TIME 20 MINUTES

Pickled veg have probiotic benefits, improving the health of your gut microbiome.

pickled vegetable salad

8 small shallots

1 small cauliflower

1 red pepper

1 litre (1 ¾ pints) water

150 ml (¼ pint) white wine vinegar

150 g (5 oz) green beans

150 g (5 oz) sugar snap peas

75 g (3 oz) watercress

olive oil

salt and pepper

Trim the shallots and break the cauliflower into small florets. Core and deseed the pepper and cut the flesh into 2 cm (¾ inch) squares.

Put the measured water and vinegar into a heavy-based saucepan, bring to the boil and add the cauliflower, pepper and shallots. Return the liquid to the boil and boil for 2 minutes. Take the saucepan off the heat and leave the vegetables to cool in the liquid.

Trim the beans and sugar snap peas and blanch in lightly salted boiling water. Refresh them in cold water and drain.

When the pickling liquid is cool, strain the vegetables and mix them with the beans, peas and watercress in a large salad bowl. Dress with olive oil, season to taste with salt and pepper and serve.

FOR PICKLED CUCUMBER & CHILLI SALAD

Cut 2 cucumbers in half lengthways and remove the seeds by running a small teaspoon along the centre. Slice the cucumber diagonally and place in a non-metallic bowl. Add 1 tablespoon finely sliced pickled ginger, 1 deseeded and finely sliced red chilli and 5 finely sliced spring onions. Put 100 g (3½ oz) sugar, 75 ml (3 fl oz) rice wine vinegar and 400 ml (14 fl oz) water in a heavy-based saucepan and bring to the boil. Allow to cool, then pour the liquid over the cucumbers and leave to stand for at least 1 hour. The pickled cucumbers will keep for up to 1 week in a covered container in the refrigerator.

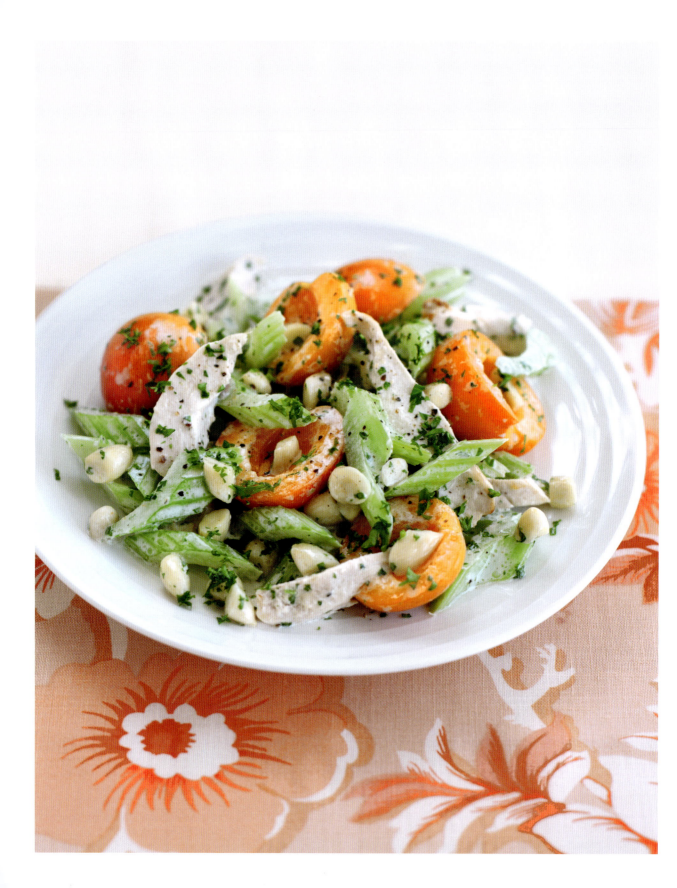

SERVES 4

PREPARATION TIME 10 MINUTES

Apricots contain carotenoids, which have anti-inflammatory potential. Choose apricots that are ripe and deep orange for the highest amount of carotenoids.

chicken, apricot & almond salad

200 g (7 oz) celery

75 g (3 oz) almonds

3 tablespoons chopped parsley

4 tablespoons mayonnaise

3 poached or roasted chicken breasts, each about 150 g (5 oz)

12 fresh apricots

salt and pepper

Thinly slice the celery sticks diagonally, reserving the yellow inner leaves. Transfer to a large salad bowl together with half the leaves. Roughly chop the almonds and add half to the bowl with the parsley and mayonnaise. Season to taste with salt and pepper.

Arrange the salad on a serving plate. Shred the chicken and halve and stone the apricots. Add the chicken and apricots to the salad and stir lightly to combine. Garnish with the remaining almonds and celery leaves and serve.

FOR GRILLED CHICKEN WITH APRICOT & TOMATO SALAD

Marinate 4 chicken breasts, each about 150 g (5 oz), with 2 crushed garlic cloves, 50 ml (2 fl oz) sweet chilli sauce and the rind and juice of 1 lime for at least 1 hour. Remove the chicken from the marinade and transfer to a heated griddle pan. Cook until golden and cooked through. Remove the stones and chop 12 apricots into 5 mm (¼ inch) pieces. Mix with 3 ripe tomatoes cut into 5 mm (¼ inch) pieces and 2 tablespoons chopped fresh coriander. Whisk together 3 tablespoons red wine vinegar, 3 tablespoons olive oil, 1 teaspoon brown sugar and 1 teaspoon soy sauce and pour the dressing over the salad. Combine well and serve with the chicken.

SERVES 4

PREPARATION TIME 15 MINUTES

> The deeper pink the watermelon, the more anti-inflammatory lycopene it contains. Be sure to mop up all the juice!

watermelon, feta & herb salad

¼ watermelon, about 800 g (1¾ lb 10 oz) in total, peeled and cut into large chunks

1 small bunch of parsley, finely chopped

1 small bunch of mint, finely chopped

1 small bunch of fresh coriander, finely chopped

200 g (7 oz) reduced-fat feta cheese, cubed

16 pitted Greek olives

1 tablespoon red jalapeño peppers in brine, drained and finely chopped

juice of 1 lime

small handful of alfalfa or radish shoots, to garnish

татьян TO SERVE

lime wedges

grissini breadsticks (optional)

Put the watermelon, herbs, feta, olives and jalapeño peppers in a large bowl and toss together.

Spoon into serving dishes and pour over the lime juice. Garnish with the alfalfa or radish shoots and serve with lime wedges and grissini breadsticks, if liked.

FOR WATERMELON FRUIT SALAD

Mix together the watermelon and chopped mint with 2 peeled, sliced kiwifruit, 200 g (7 oz) halved red grapes, 2 small, peeled, cored and thinly sliced apples and 200 g (7 oz) pitted cherries, if in season. Dust with a little icing sugar, if liked, and squeeze over the lime juice. Serve chilled.

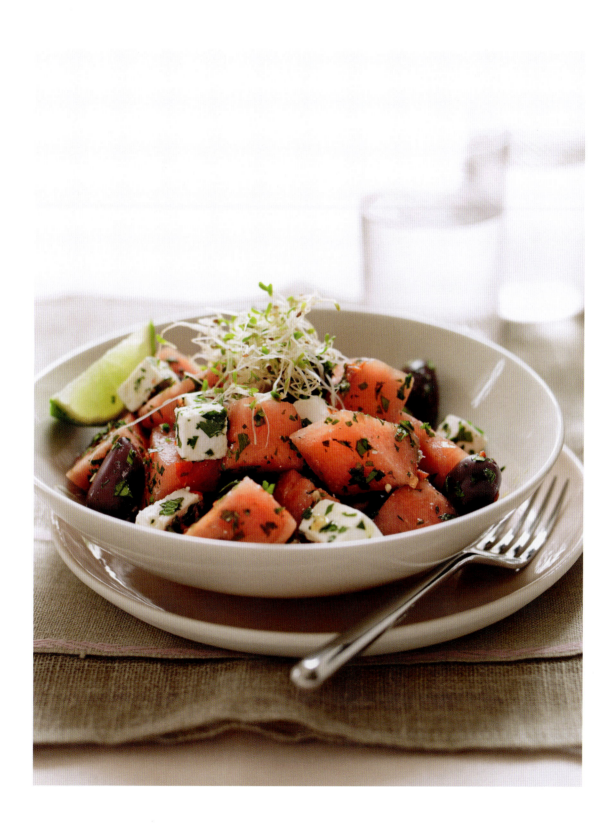

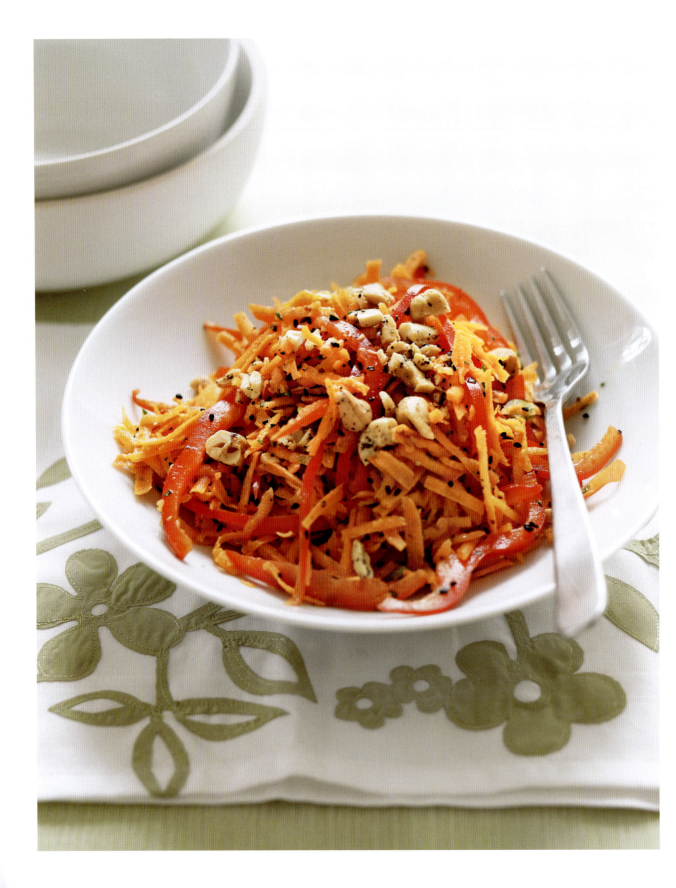

SERVES 4

PREPARATION TIME 10 MINUTES

COOKING TIME 6–10 MINUTES

Cashews provide plenty of iron, which keeps red blood cells healthy and protects against low energy levels.

carrot & cashew nut salad

75 g (3 oz) unsalted cashew nuts

2 tablespoons black mustard seeds

500 g (1 lb) carrots, peeled and coarsely grated

1 red pepper, cored, deseeded and thinly sliced

3 tablespoons chopped chervil

2 spring onions, finely sliced

DRESSING

2 tablespoons avocado oil

2 tablespoons raspberry vinegar

1 tablespoon wholegrain mustard

pinch of sugar

salt and pepper

Heat a nonstick frying pan over a medium-low heat and dry-fry the cashew nuts for 5–8 minutes, stirring frequently, or until golden brown and toasted. Tip on to a small plate and leave to cool. Add the mustard seeds to the pan and dry-fry for 1–2 minutes or until they start to pop.

Mix together the mustard seeds, carrots, red pepper, chervil and spring onions in a large bowl.

Whisk together all the dressing ingredients in a small bowl, then pour over the grated carrot salad. Mix thoroughly to coat and heap into serving bowls.

Chop the cashew nuts coarsely and scatter them over the salad. Serve immediately.

FOR CARROT & CELERIAC COLESLAW

Mix together 300 g (10 oz) grated carrot and 200 g (7 oz) coarsely grated celeriac with the mustard seeds, chervil, spring onions and dressing, omitting the red pepper. Replace the cashew nuts with 75 g (3 oz) chopped walnuts and serve as above.

SERVES 4

PREPARATION TIME 10 MINUTES, PLUS COOLING

COOKING TIME 20 MINUTES

> Chia seeds add extra plant protein, omega-3s and fibre to this dish, making it a nutritionally balanced light lunch.

Mediterranean potato salad

450 g (14½ oz) potatoes, peeled and cut into chunks

pinch of saffron threads

125 g (4 oz) sunblush tomatoes, halved

75 g (3 oz) pitted black olives, roughly chopped

6 tablespoons olive oil

4 tablespoons chia seeds

5 tablespoons chopped basil leaves

3 tablespoons capers

salt and pepper

fresh crusty bread or rocket salad, to serve (optional)

Pour over just enough cold water to cover the potatoes in a saucepan and add the saffron. Bring to the boil, then cover and simmer very gently for 15 minutes until tender and cooked through. Drain and leave to cool.

Put the sunblush tomatoes, olives, oil, chia seeds, basil leaves and capers in a large bowl, add the cooled potatoes and gently toss together. Season with a little salt and plenty of pepper.

Divide the salad between 4 serving bowls and serve with fresh crusty bread or a simple rocket salad if liked.

FOR MEDITERRANEAN PASTA SALAD

Cook 225 g (7½ oz) dried pasta shapes in a large saucepan of lightly salted boiling water for 8–10 minutes until just tender. Drain well, rinse under cold water and drain again. Put 125 g (4 oz) roughly chopped sunblush tomatoes, 75 g (3 oz) roughly chopped pitted black olives, 6 tablespoons olive oil, 4 tablespoons chia seeds, 5 tablespoons chopped basil leaves and 3 tablespoons capers in a large bowl. Toss well so that all the ingredients are well mixed. Season with salt and pepper before serving.

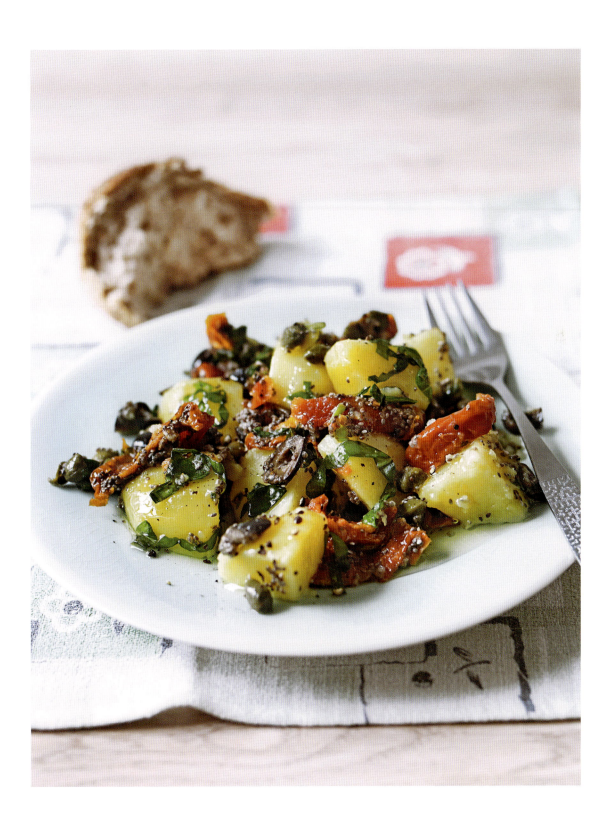

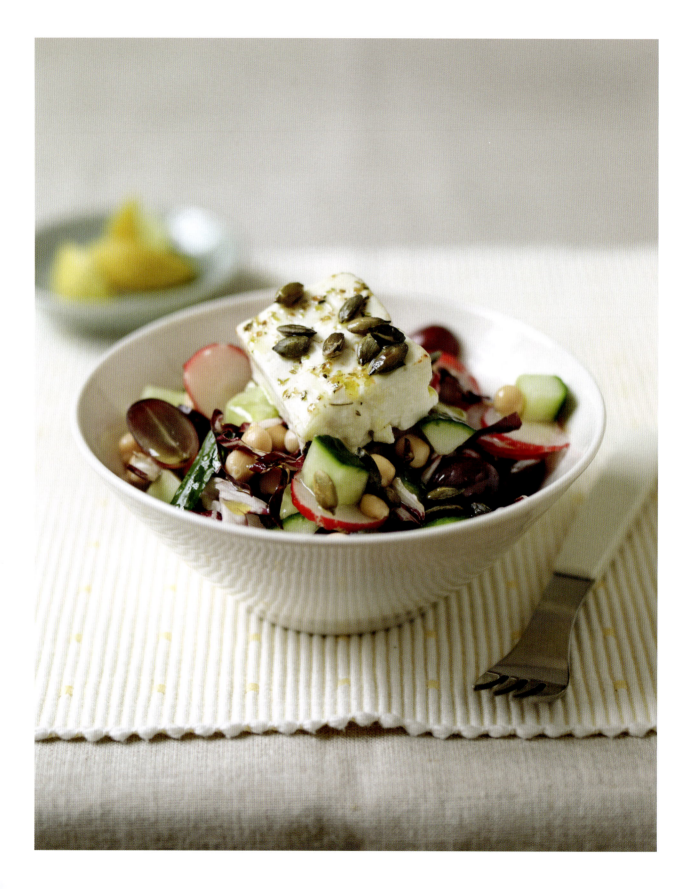

SERVES 4

PREPARATION TIME 10 MINUTES

COOKING TIME 5–7 MINUTES

chickpea & feta salad

400 g (13 oz) can chickpeas, drained

1 Lebanese cucumber or ½ cucumber, diced

150 g (5 oz) radishes, thinly sliced

150 g (5 oz) red seedless grapes, halved

1 small radicchio, sliced

200 g (7 oz) reduced-fat feta cheese, cut into 4 pieces

2 tablespoons extra virgin rapeseed or olive oil

½ teaspoon dried oregano

2 heaped tablespoons pumpkin seeds

small handful of radish sprouts (optional)

salt and pepper

lemon wedges, to serve

Mix together the chickpeas, cucumber, radishes and grapes in a large bowl. Toss lightly with the radicchio, season with salt and pepper and pile into serving dishes.

Place the feta on a foil-lined grill pan, drizzle with 2 teaspoons of the oil and sprinkle with the dried oregano and a little pepper. Cook under a preheated hot grill for 3–4 minutes or until golden. Remove from the grill and leave to cool for 2–3 minutes.

Meanwhile, heat a small nonstick frying pan over a medium heat, add the pumpkin seeds and dry-fry for 2–3 minutes or until lightly golden. Tip on to a small plate.

Arrange the grilled feta on the salad. Scatter over the toasted pumpkin seeds and radish sprouts, if using. Drizzle with the remaining oil and serve immediately with the lemon wedges.

FOR WATERMELON & HALLOUMI SALAD

Mix together ½ peeled watermelon, cut into large chunks, with 2 tablespoons chopped mint, ½ finely chopped red onion, 16–20 pitted black olives and the chickpeas. Replace the feta with 200 g (7 oz) halloumi cheese and cut into slices. Brush with the oil and grill as above. Serve with the pumpkin seeds as above.

SERVES 4
PREPARATION TIME 10 MINUTES
COOKING TIME 40–45 MINUTES

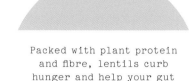

Packed with plant protein and fibre, lentils curb hunger and help your gut microbiome to thrive.

warm lentil, tomato & onion salad

1 tablespoon olive oil

1 large red onion, thinly sliced

50 g (2 oz) fresh root ginger, peeled and chopped

4 garlic cloves, thinly sliced

125 g (4 oz) green lentils, rinsed

100 g (3½ oz) red lentils, rinsed

½ teaspoon ground cinnamon

400 g (13 oz) tomatoes, roughly chopped, or 400 g (13 oz) can chopped tomatoes

350 ml (12 fl oz) water or vegetable stock

2 teaspoons nigella seeds

salt and pepper

parsley, to garnish

TO SERVE

lemon wedges

wholemeal flatbreads (optional)

Heat the oil in a large, heavy-based saucepan over a medium-low heat, add the onion, ginger and garlic and cook gently for 10 minutes until softened but not coloured.

Stir in the lentils and cinnamon. Add the tomatoes and measured water or stock. Season with salt and pepper and bring to the boil. Reduce the heat, cover and leave to simmer gently for 30–35 minutes or until the lentils are tender and the liquid has been absorbed.

Spoon the lentils into bowls, sprinkle with the nigella seeds and garnish with parsley leaves. Serve warm with lemon wedges and toasted wholemeal flatbreads, if liked.

FOR NO-COOK LENTIL, TOMATO & ONION SALAD

Rinse and drain a 250 g (8 oz) pack cooked lentils. Place in a bowl and mix with ½ finely chopped red onion, 4 chopped tomatoes, 1 small crushed garlic clove, a 1 cm (½ inch) piece of peeled and finely grated fresh root ginger and 2 tablespoons chopped parsley. Make a dressing with 1 tablespoon olive oil, 2 tablespoons lemon juice, pinch of ground cinnamon, pinch of ground paprika and some salt and pepper. Toss the lentil salad in the dressing and serve, garnished, as above.

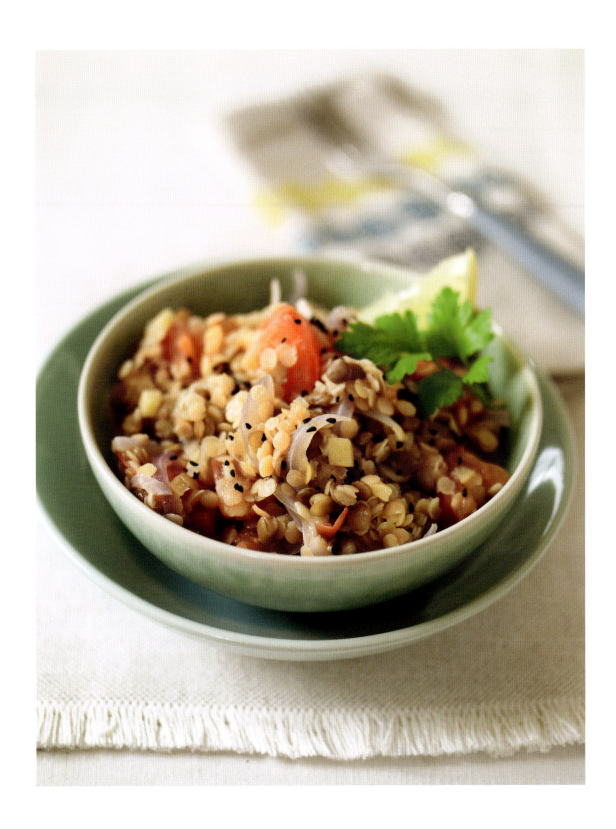

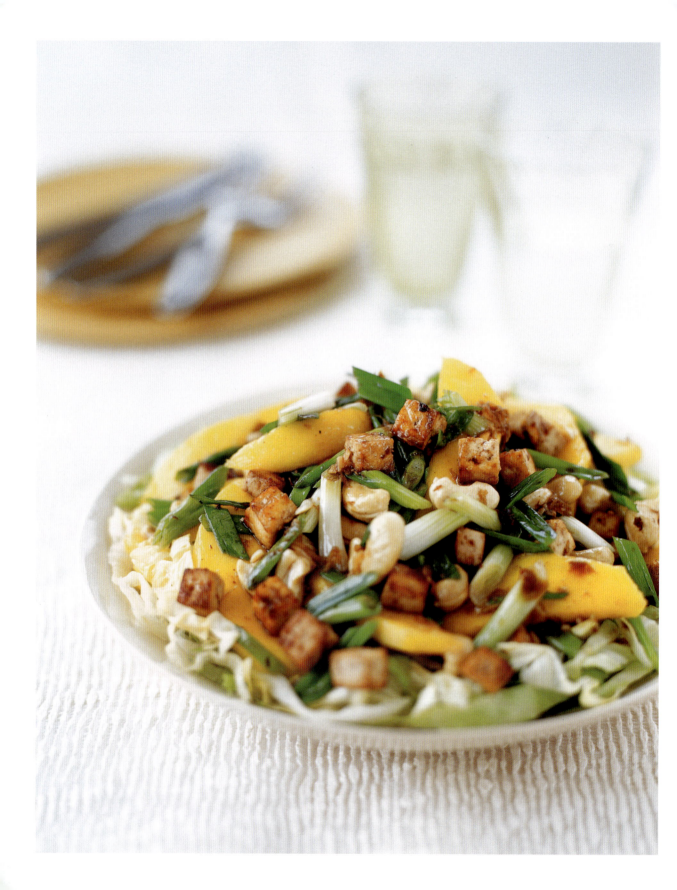

SERVES 2

PREPARATION TIME 15 MINUTES, PLUS MARINATING

COOKING TIME 5 MINUTES

> Ginger is rich in anti-inflammatory components called gingerols and shogaols.

gingered tofu & mango salad

25 g (1 oz) fresh root ginger, peeled and grated

2 tablespoons light soy sauce

1 garlic clove, finely chopped

1 tablespoon seasoned rice vinegar

125 g (4 oz) firm silken tofu, cut into 1 cm (½ inch) cubes

2 tablespoons groundnut or vegetable oil

1 bunch of spring onions, sliced diagonally into 1.5 cm (¾ inch) lengths

40 g (1½ oz) cashew nuts

1 small mango, peeled, stoned and sliced

½ small iceberg lettuce, shredded

Mix together the ginger, soy sauce, garlic and vinegar in a small bowl. Add the tofu to the bowl and toss the ingredients together. Leave to marinate for 15 minutes.

Lift the tofu from the marinade with a fork, drain it and reserve the marinade. Heat the oil in a frying pan over a medium heat, add the tofu pieces and gently fry for 3 minutes or until golden. Remove with a slotted spoon and keep warm.

Add the spring onions and cashew nuts to the pan and fry quickly for 30 seconds. Add the mango slices to the pan and cook for 30 seconds or until heated through.

Pile the lettuce on to serving plates and scatter the tofu, spring onions, mango and cashew nuts over the top. Heat the marinade juices in the pan with 2 tablespoons water, pour the mixture over the salad and serve immediately.

FOR TOFU & SUGAR SNAP SALAD

Marinate and fry the tofu as above. Add the spring onions and cashew nuts to the pan, also adding 1 red chilli, sliced into rounds, and 100 g (3½ oz) halved sugar snap peas. Omit the mango. Fry for 1 minute until heated through, then gently toss in the fried tofu. Add the juice of ½ lime and 2 tablespoons water to the reserved marinade and drizzle it over the salad before serving on the lettuce.

SERVES 2

PREPARATION TIME 10–15 MINUTES

Greek-style salad

½ cucumber

4 plum tomatoes

1 red pepper

1 green pepper

½ red onion

60 g (2¼ oz) pitted Kalamata olives

50 g (2 oz) feta cheese, diced

DRESSING

4 tablespoons olive oil

1 tablespoon chopped parsley

salt and pepper

Cut the cucumber and tomatoes into 1–2 cm (½–¾ inch) chunks and put them in a large salad bowl. Cut the flesh from the peppers and carefully remove the ribs and the seeds. Cut the pepper flesh into thin strips and put them in the bowl with the cucumber and tomatoes. Finely slice the red onion and add to the bowl with the olives.

Make the dressing by whisking the oil and parsley together. Season to taste with salt and pepper.

Pour the dressing over the salad and toss carefully. Transfer to serving bowls, scatter some feta evenly over each bowl and serve.

FOR GREEK-STYLE SALAD WITH GARLIC PITTA BREAD

Rub 4 pitta breads with a peeled clove of garlic, drizzle with olive oil, season with salt and pepper and toast in a preheated oven, 190°C (375°F), Gas Mark 5, for 4–5 minutes until crisp. Roughly break the pitta breads into pieces, about 2 cm (¾ inch) square, and set aside. Prepare the Greek-style Salad as above, adding 2 tablespoons chopped basil and 2 tablespoons chopped mint. Toss the salad and serve, garnished with the pitta bread pieces and a dollop of hummus on each plate.

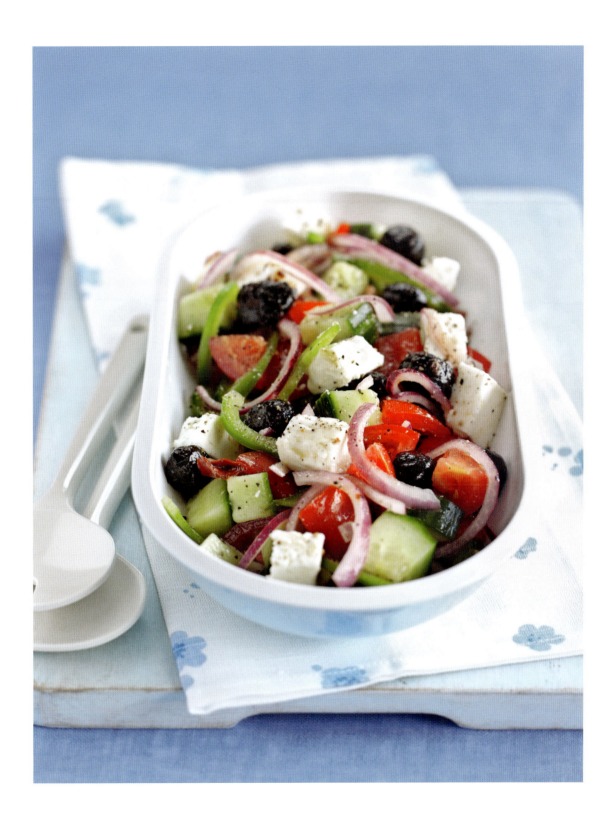

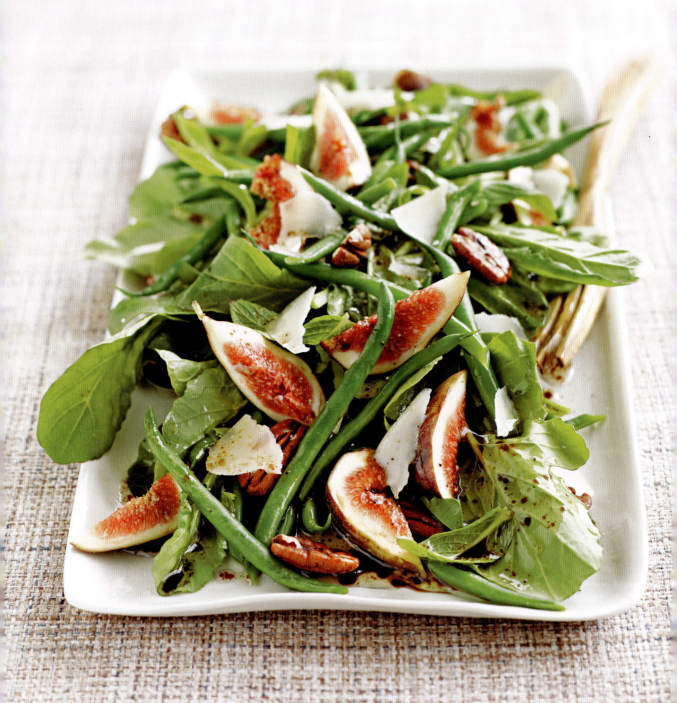

SERVES 4

PREPARATION TIME 5 MINUTES, PLUS COOLING

COOKING TIME 5–6 MINUTES

Figs contain a range of flavonoids and phenolic acids that help reduce oxidation and inflammation.

fig, bean & toasted pecan salad

100 g (3½ oz) pecan nuts

200 g (7 oz) green beans, trimmed

4 fresh figs, cut into quarters

100 g (3½ oz) baby leaf salad

small handful of mint leaves

50 g (2 oz) Parmesan or pecorino cheese

DRESSING

3 tablespoons walnut oil

2 teaspoons sherry vinegar

1 teaspoon vincotto or balsamic vinegar

salt and pepper

Heat a heavy-based frying pan over a medium heat, add the pecan nuts and dry-fry, stirring frequently, for 3–4 minutes or until browned. Tip on to a small plate and leave to cool.

Cook the beans in a saucepan of lightly salted boiling water for 2 minutes. Drain, refresh under running cold water and pat dry with kitchen paper. Put the beans in a bowl with the figs, pecan nuts, salad leaves and mint.

Whisk together all the dressing ingredients in a small bowl and season with salt and paper. Pour over the salad and toss well. Shave over the Parmesan or pecorino and serve.

FOR MIXED BEAN SALAD

Combine 200 g (7 oz) cooked trimmed green beans with 2 x 400 g (13 oz) cans drained mixed beans, 4 finely chopped spring onions, 1 crushed garlic clove and 4 tablespoons chopped mixed herbs, then dress with 4 tablespoons olive oil, juice of ½ lemon, a pinch of caster sugar and salt and pepper.

SERVES 4

PREPARATION TIME 15 MINUTES, PLUS STANDING

panzanella-style salad

600 g (1¼ lb) large tomatoes

1 tablespoon sea salt

150 g (5 oz) ciabatta

½ red onion, finely chopped

1 handful of basil leaves, plus extra to garnish

1 tablespoon red wine vinegar

2 tablespoons olive oil

12 pickled white anchovies, drained

salt and pepper

Roughly chop the tomatoes into 2 cm (¾ inch) pieces and put them in a non-metallic bowl. Sprinkle over the sea salt and leave to stand for 1 hour.

Remove the crusts from the ciabatta and tear the bread into rough chunks.

Give the tomatoes a good squash with clean hands, then add the bread, onion, basil, vinegar and oil. Season to taste with salt and pepper. Mix together carefully and transfer to serving plates. Garnish with the drained anchovies and extra basil and serve.

FOR TOMATO & BEAN SALAD

Finely slice 1 red onion, cover with 4 tablespoons red wine vinegar and leave to stand for about 30 minutes. Cut 150 g (5 oz) ciabatta bread into chunks and place in a roasting tin. Drizzle with olive oil, season with salt and pepper and add 2 sprigs of thyme. Cook the ciabatta in a preheated oven, 190°C (375°F), Gas Mark 5, until golden and crispy. Dice 300 g (10 oz) tomatoes and put them in a large bowl. Add 410 g (13½ oz) can borlotti beans, rinsed and drained, 410 g (13½ oz) can cannellini beans, rinsed and drained, and 1 bunch of chopped basil. Remove the onion from the vinegar, reserving the vinegar, and add to the salad with 12 drained pickled white anchovies. Add 1 teaspoon Dijon mustard to the reserved vinegar and whisk in 5 tablespoons olive oil. Season with salt and pepper. Add the dressing to the salad, toss thoroughly and serve, garnished with the ciabatta croûtons.

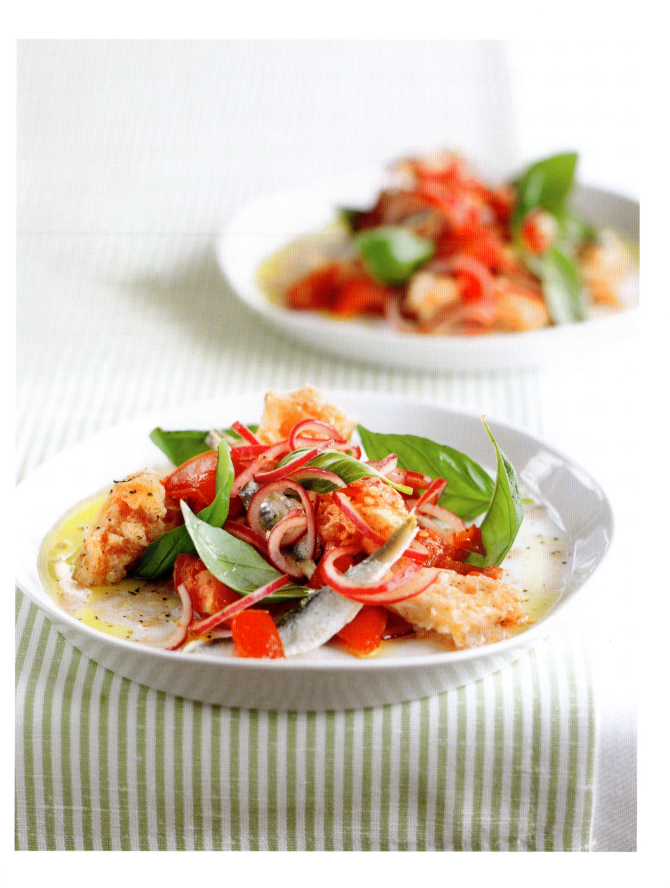

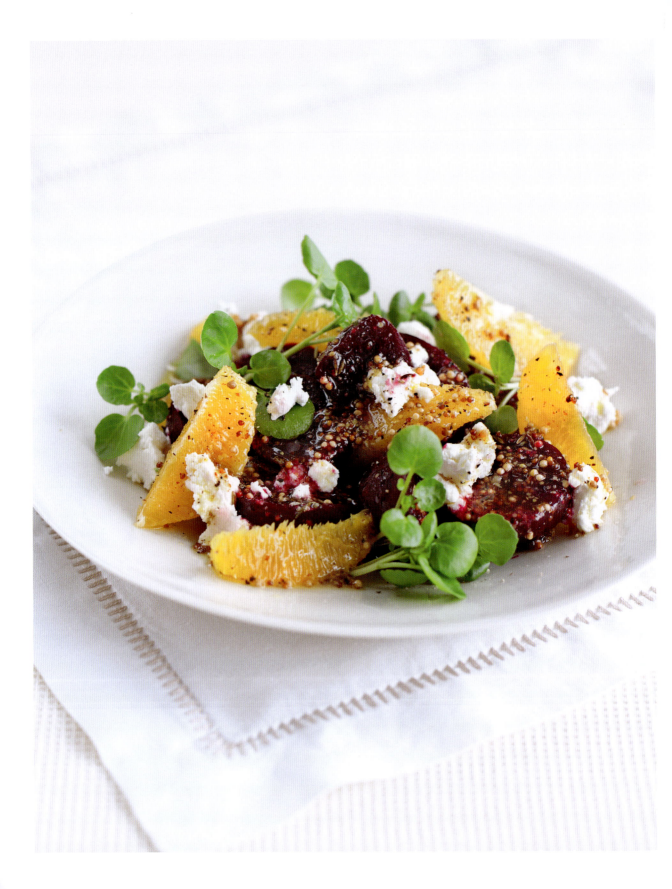

SERVES 2—4
PREPARATION TIME 15 MINUTES
COOKING TIME 30 MINUTES

Beetroot is a natural source of nitrates, which can improve blood flow and lower blood pressure.

beetroot & orange salad

7 small beetroot

1 teaspoon cumin seeds

1 tablespoon red wine vinegar

2 oranges

65 g (2½ oz) watercress

75 g (3 oz) soft goats' cheese

DRESSING

1 tablespoon clear honey

1 teaspoon wholegrain mustard

1 ½ tablespoons white wine vinegar

3 tablespoons olive oil

salt and pepper

Scrub and trim the beetroot and put them in a foil-lined roasting tin with the cumin seeds and vinegar and bake in a preheated oven, 190°C (375°F), Gas Mark 5, for 30 minutes or until cooked. Check by piercing one with a knife. Allow the beetroot to cool slightly and then, wearing food-handling gloves, rub off the skin and slice the globes into halves, or quarters if large.

Meanwhile, peel and segment the oranges. Make the dressing by whisking together the honey, mustard, vinegar and oil. Season to taste with salt and pepper.

Put the watercress in a bowl with the beetroot and add the dressing. Mix gently to combine. Arrange the oranges on a plate, top with the salad and crumble over the cheese. Season with pepper and serve.

SERVES 4

PREPARATION TIME 20 MINUTES, PLUS MARINATING

COOKING TIME 20 MINUTES

> Pomegranates and pomegranate extracts have been shown to decrease markers of inflammation in the body.

chicken couscous salad

4 boneless, skinless chicken breasts, each about 125 g (4 oz)

300 g (10 oz) wholemeal couscous

300 ml (½ pint) hot chicken stock

1 pomegranate

rind and juice of 1 orange

1 small bunch of fresh coriander

1 small bunch of mint

FOR THE MARINADE

1½ tablespoons curry paste (tikka masala)

5 tablespoons natural yogurt

1 teaspoon olive oil

2 tablespoons lemon juice

Make the marinade by mixing together the curry paste, yogurt and oil. Put the chicken in a non-metallic dish, cover with half the marinade and leave for at least 1 hour.

Put the couscous in a bowl, add the hot stock, cover and leave for 8 minutes.

Meanwhile, cut the pomegranate in half and remove the seeds. Add them to the couscous with the orange rind and juice.

Remove the chicken from the marinade, reserving the marinade, and transfer to a foil-lined baking sheet. Cook in a preheated oven, 190°C (375°F), Gas Mark 5, for 6–7 minutes, then transfer to a preheated hot grill and cook for 2 minutes until caramelized. Cover with foil and leave to rest for 5 minutes.

Roughly chop the coriander and mint, reserving some whole coriander leaves for garnish, and add to the couscous. Thinly slice the chicken. Spoon the couscous on to plates and add the chicken. Thin the reserved marinade with the lemon juice and drizzle over the couscous. Garnish with the reserved coriander leaves and serve immediately.

FOR POMEGRANATE VINAIGRETTE

Whisk together 150 ml (¼ pint) pomegranate juice, 2 tablespoons pomegranate molasses (available from Middle Eastern stores and some supermarkets), 2 tablespoons red wine vinegar and 3 tablespoons olive oil. Use to dress the salad instead of the reserved marinade.

SERVES 4

PREPARATION TIME 15 MINUTES

COOKING TIME 5 MINUTES

spiced chicken & mango salad

4 boneless, skinless chicken breasts, about 150 g (5 oz) each

6 teaspoons mild curry paste

4 tablespoons lemon juice

150 ml (¼ pint) natural yogurt

50 g (2 oz) watercress

½ cucumber, diced

½ red onion, finely choppes

1 mango, peeled, stoned and cut into chunks

½ iceberg lettuce

Cut the chicken breasts into long, thin slices. Put 4 teaspoons of the curry paste in a plastic bag with the lemon juice and mix together by squeezing the bag. Add the chicken and toss together.

Half-fill the base of a steamer with water and bring to the boil. Steam the chicken in a single layer, covered, for 5 minutes until cooked. Test with a knife or metal skewer; the juices will run clear when it is done.

Meanwhile, mix the remaining curry paste in a bowl with the yogurt.

Tear the watercress into bite-sized pieces. Add it to the yogurt dressing with the cucumber, red onion and mango and toss gently.

Tear the lettuce into pieces and arrange on 4 plates. Spoon the mango mixture over the top, add the warm chicken strips and serve immediately.

FOR CHILLI PRAWN, MANGO & AVOCADO SALAD

Replace the chicken with 400 g (13 oz) peeled, raw tiger prawns with the tails on. Prepare the salad in the same way as above but add the diced flesh of an avocado. Heat 2 tablespoons vegetable or groundnut oil in a nonstick frying pan over a high heat, and fry 1 finely chopped red chilli for 1 minute, then add the prawns and 2 finely chopped garlic cloves. Fry for 2 minutes until the prawns are pink and just cooked through. Mix through the salad and serve immediately.

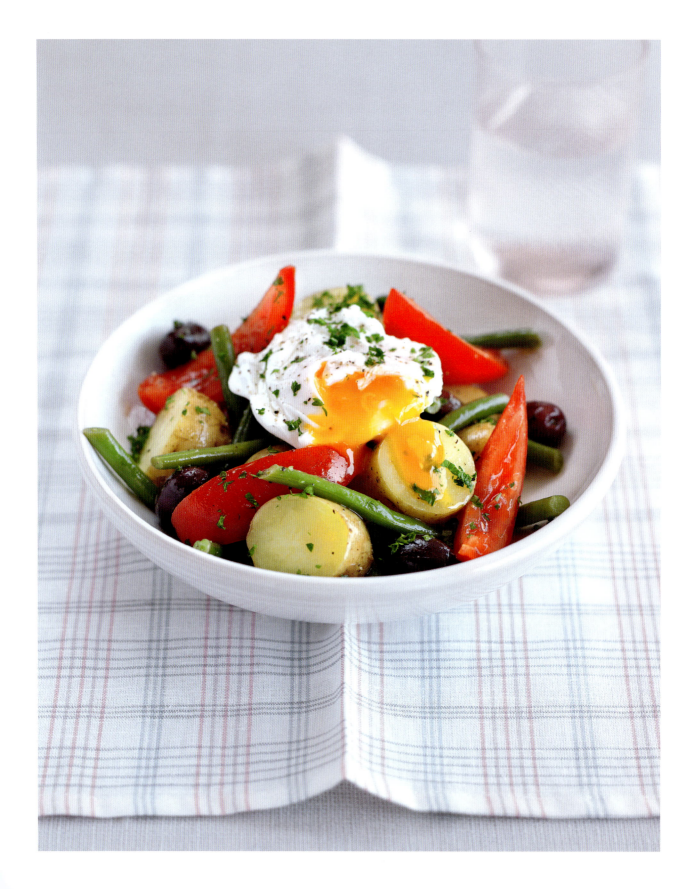

SERVES 4
PREPARATION TIME 15 MINUTES
COOKING TIME 10–15 MINUTES

Niçoise salad

400 g (13 oz) small potatoes

200 g (7 oz) green beans, trimmed

5 large plum tomatoes

2 tablespoons chopped parsley, plus extra leaves to garnish

60 g (2¼ oz) pitted black olives

2 tablespoons lemon juice

2–3 tablespoons olive oil

4 soft-poached large eggs

salt and pepper

Cook the potatoes in lightly salted boiling water, leave them to cool and halve them. Meanwhile, bring a large saucepan of lightly salted water to the boil, add the trimmed green beans and blanch for 1–2 minutes until bright green and still firm to the touch. Refresh in cold water, drain and transfer to a large salad bowl.

Core the tomatoes and cut each one into 6 pieces. Add the tomatoes and chopped parsley to the beans with the potatoes, olives, lemon juice and oil. Season to taste with salt and pepper.

Transfer the salad to serving plates and top each one with a poached egg cut in half and a drizzle of olive oil. Garnish with the extra parsley leaves and serve.

FOR TUNA NIÇOISE SALAD

Prepare the salad in the same way as the Niçoise salad. Drain 185 g (6¼ oz) canned tuna in olive oil. Flake the fish and toss it through the Niçoise salad and serve, topped with a soft-poached egg, if liked.

Snacks & Starters

89	**baby green peppers in olive oil**
90	**guacamole with pickled ginger**
93	**chilli, lime & coriander dried fruit & nuts**
94	**tandoori tofu bites**
96	**herb oatcakes**
97	**smoked mackerel crostini**
98	**pea & mint falafel with mint dip**
101	**cheat's Mediterranean focaccia**
102	**harissa & tahini hummus**
105	**bruschetta with tomatoes & ricotta**
106	**parsnip & beetroot crisps with homemade dukkah**
109	**aubergine dip with flatbreads**
110	**ricotta-stuffed mushrooms**
113	**courgette, beetroot & feta fritters**
114	**chicken bites with salsa**
116	**bean, lemon & rosemary hummus**
117	**smashed bean & sardine dip**
118	**vegetable kebabs with harissa yogurt**

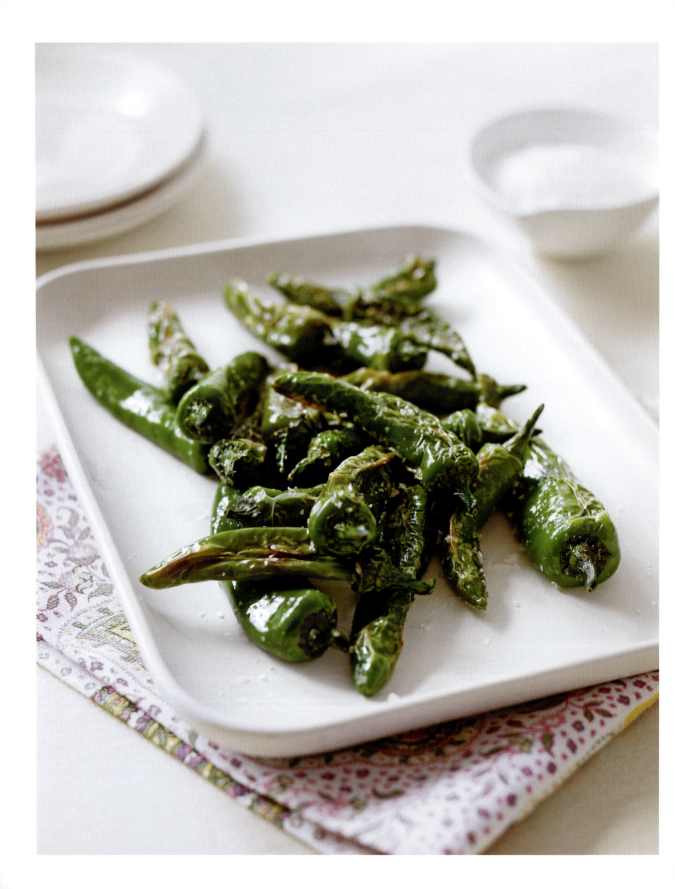

SERVES 6
PREPARATION TIME 5 MINUTES
COOKING TIME 3–5 MINUTES

A true taste of the Mediterranean, this Padron pepper dish is rich in anti-inflammatory vitamin C and monounsaturates.

baby green peppers in olive oil

3 tablespoons olive oil

250 g (8 oz) Padrón peppers or baby green peppers, or mild green chillies

flaky sea salt

Heat the oil in a large frying pan, add the peppers or chillies and cook over a high heat for 3–5 minutes, turning frequently, until the skins start to brown.

Remove from the pan and drain on kitchen paper, then serve scattered with flaky sea salt.

FOR CHARRED GREEN PEPPER TOASTS

Cook the peppers as above, then leave to cool. Halve the peppers and discard the seeds, membranes and stalks, then cut into chunks. Toss together with 3 chopped tomatoes and 50 g (2 oz) chopped pitted olives in a bowl. Whisk together 1 crushed garlic clove, 1 tablespoon red wine vinegar and 3 tablespoons olive oil in a small bowl. Stir into the pepper mixture along with a handful of chopped parsley. Halve 6 large slices of country-style bread, drizzle with olive oil and toast under a preheated hot grill until lightly browned. Spoon the pepper mixture on top of the toasts and serve.

SERVES 4

PREPARATION TIME 15 MINUTES

guacamole with pickled ginger

2 ripe avocados

juice of 2 small limes

1–2 teaspoons wasabi paste, to taste

4 spring onions, finely chopped

1 tablespoon sesame seeds, toasted

1 teaspoon Japanese rice mirin

1 teaspoon finely chopped pickled ginger

sesame seeds, for sprinkling

prawn or rice crackers, to serve

Cut the avocados in half and remove and discard the stones. Peel off the skin and roughly chop the flesh. Place in a bowl and roughly mash with a fork.

Stir in the lime juice, wasabi, spring onions, sesame seeds and mirin.

Transfer to a serving bowl and scatter over the pickled ginger and sesame seeds. Serve immediately, with crackers for dipping.

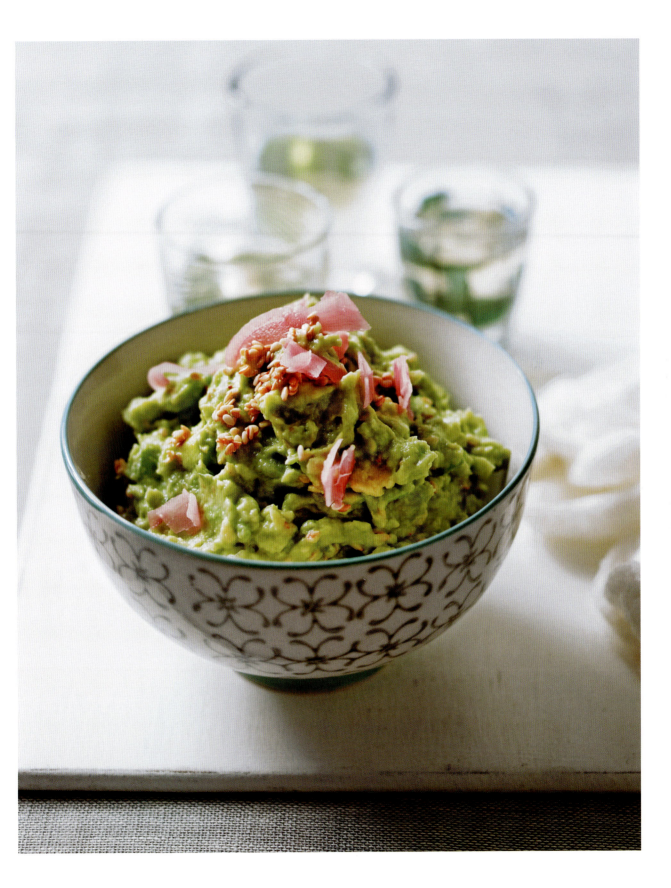

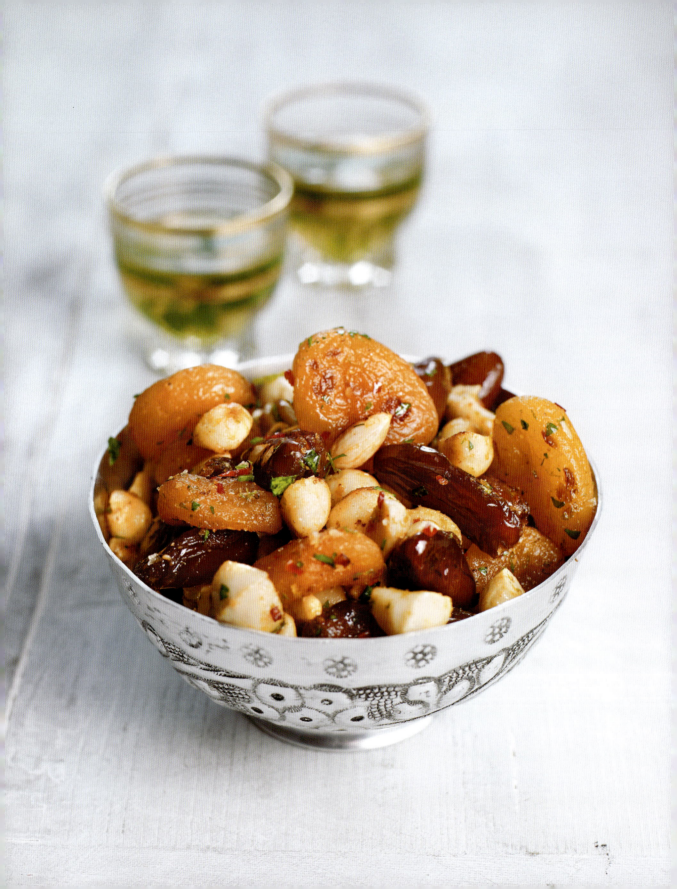

SERVES 4

PREPARATION TIME 5 MINUTES

COOKING TIME 6–8 MINUTES

> Containing fibre and minerals alongside the natural sugars, dried fruit is a healthy way to satisfy sweet cravings.

chilli, lime & coriander dried fruit & nuts

120 g (4 oz) whole almonds

2 tablespoons olive oil

2 tablespoons macadamia nuts, halved

2 tablespoons cashew nuts, halved

120 g (4 oz) ready-to-eat dried apricots

120 g (4 oz) ready-to-eat pitted dates

1–2 teaspoons finely chopped dried red chilli

grated rind of 1 lime

1 small bunch of fresh coriander, finely chopped

salt

Put the almonds in a bowl and pour over enough boiling water to cover. Leave for 5 minutes, then drain, refresh under cold running water and drain again. Using your fingers, rub the skins off the almonds and cut in half.

Heat the olive oil in a large, heavy-based frying pan, add the nuts and dried fruit and cook, stirring, for 4–5 minutes until the nuts begin to colour. Toss in the chilli and lime rind and cook for a further 2–3 minutes, then season with salt and add the coriander. Serve immediately.

SERVES 4

PREPARATION TIME 15 MINUTES, PLUS STANDING AND MARINATING

COOKING TIME 20–25 MINUTES

> Firm tofu coagulated with nigari (check the label) is a rich source of magnesium, which is needed for healthy muscles and nerves.

tandoori tofu bites

400 g (13 oz) firm tofu, drained

MARINADE

100 ml (3½ fl oz) thick natural yogurt

1 teaspoon peeled and grated fresh root ginger

1 garlic clove, crushed

1 tablespoon tandoori masala

1 teaspoon garam masala

1 teaspoon ground coriander

½ teaspoon salt

¼ teaspoon ground turmeric

2 tablespoons lemon juice

TO SERVE

lemon wedges

sprigs of parsley

Place the tofu between 2 pieces of kitchen paper and set a chopping board or other weight on top. Leave to stand for at least 10 minutes to remove the excess water.

Remove the weight and kitchen paper, then cut the tofu into cubes.

Mix all the marinade ingredients together in a large non-metallic bowl and stir in the tofu. Cover and leave to marinate for 1 hour.

Place the tofu pieces on a lightly oiled nonstick baking sheet and cook in a preheated oven, 200°C (400°F), Gas Mark 6, for 20–25 minutes, turning halfway through the cooking time.

Serve the tofu cubes with cocktail sticks for skewering, lemon wedges and a parsley garnish.

FOR BAKED TERIYAKI TOFU BITES

Follow the recipe above to remove the excess water from the tofu, then cut into cubes. For the marinade, mix together 2 tablespoons each of dark soy sauce and rice wine or dry sherry, 2 teaspoons peeled and chopped fresh root ginger, 1 teaspoon chopped garlic and 1 tablespoon each of soft light brown sugar and sesame seeds in a large non-metallic bowl. Stir in the tofu, cover and leave to marinate for 30 minutes. Cook the tofu as above, then serve on cocktail sticks, garnished with shredded spring onions.

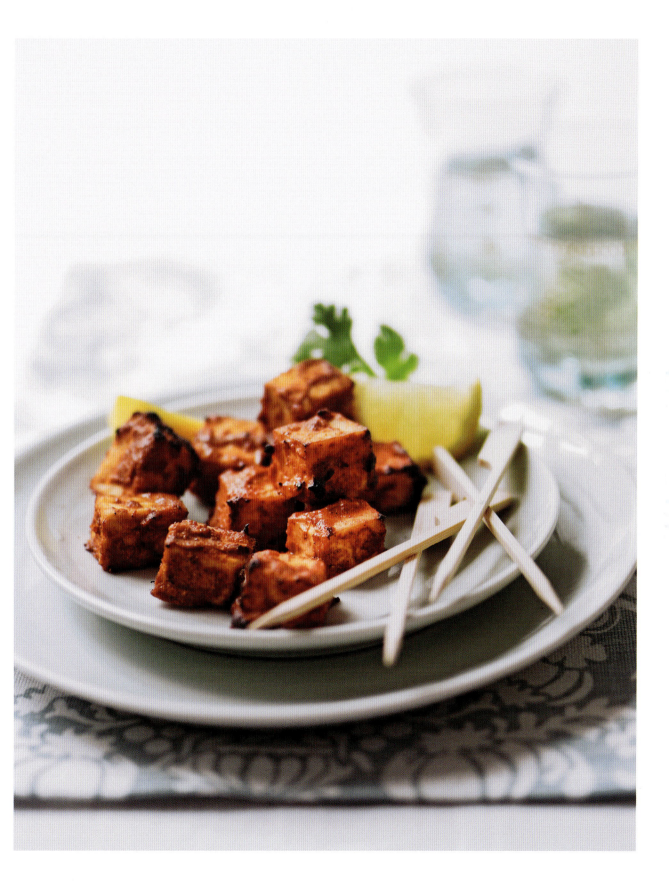

SERVES 4
PREPARATION TIME 15 MINUTES
COOKING TIME 12–15 MINUTES

> Oats contain beta glucan which can help in lowering cholesterol, as well as moderating your blood sugar levels.

herb oatcakes

200 g (7 oz) rolled oats

3 sprigs rosemary, leaves picked

125 g (4 oz) plain flour, plus extra for dusting

1 teaspoon baking powder

pinch of salt

75 g (3 oz) unsalted butter, cubed

100 ml (3½ fl oz) milk

TO SERVE

cheese of your choice

sliced apples

Place the oats and the rosemary in a food processor and process until they start to break down and the mixture resembles breadcrumbs.

Add the flour, baking powder and salt and blitz again.

Add the butter and process until it is mixed in, then pour in the milk while the machine is running and process until the dough comes together in a ball.

Turn out on to a lightly floured work surface and roll out to a thickness of about 4–5 mm (¼ inch). Cut out 20–24 rounds using a 4–5 cm (2 inch) cutter, rerolling as necessary, and place on a baking sheet.

Bake in a preheated oven, 190°C (375°F), Gas Mark 5, for 12–15 minutes until just starting to turn golden at the edges.

Cool on a wire rack and serve with cheese and apples. Store in an airtight container.

SERVES 4
PREPARATION TIME 10 MINUTES
COOKING TIME 2–3 MINUTES

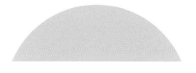

Mackerel is one of the very richest natural sources of anti-inflammatory omega-3 fats.

smoked mackerel crostini

230 g (7½ oz) smoked mackerel fillets, skinned

1 tablespoon creamed horseradish

2 tablespoons half-fat crème fraîche

1 tablespoon chopped chives

finely grated rind of 1 lemon

1 tablespoon lemon juice

1 granary or seeded baguette, sliced

1 spring onion, finely sliced diagonally (optional)

4 little gem lettuces, leaves separated

pepper

Put the smoked mackerel in a bowl and break into flakes with a fork. Add the horseradish, crème fraîche, chives, lemon rind and juice and plenty of pepper and mix together gently.

Place the sliced baguette on a grill pan and cook under a preheated medium-hot grill for 2–3 minutes or until crisp and golden, turning once. Serve the hot crostini immediately with the smoked mackerel rillettes, spring onion, if liked, and the lettuce leaves.

FOR SMOKED MACKEREL FISHCAKES

Mix the flaked mackerel with 230 g (7½ oz) cold mashed potato, 1½ tablespoons horseradish, the chives, lemon rind and pepper, omitting the crème fraîche and lemon juice. Chill for 1 hour. Form into 4 patties with slightly damp hands, then dust in flour. Blitz the baguette in a food processor or blender to make breadcrumbs. Dip each fishcake in beaten egg and coat in the breadcrumbs. Heat a little extra virgin rapeseed oil in a frying pan, add the fishcakes and fry for 4–5 minutes on each side or until cooked through and crisp. Drain on kitchen paper and serve with mixed salad leaves.

SERVES 4

PREPARATION TIME 20 MINUTES, PLUS CHILLING

COOKING TIME 5–7 MINUTES

Frozen peas are packed with thiamin, a B vitamin needed for healthy heart function and the release of energy from food.

pea & mint falafel with mint dip

175 g (6 oz) frozen peas

400 g (13 oz) can chickpeas, drained and rinsed, then drained again well

25 g (1 oz) fresh white breadcrumbs

1 garlic clove, crushed

1 red or green chilli, deseeded and finely chopped

1 tablespoon ground cumin

1 teaspoon ground coriander

4 tablespoons chopped mint

1 teaspoon baking powder

1 egg, lightly beaten

2 tablespoons sunflower oil

salt and pepper

wholemeal pitta breads, to serve

MINT DIP

100 ml (3½ fl oz) low-fat natural yogurt

2 tablespoons chopped mint

¼ cucumber, finely chopped

Cook the peas in a saucepan of boiling water for 1 minute. Drain the peas, then refresh under cold running water and drain again thoroughly.

Place the peas in a food processor with the chickpeas, breadcrumbs, garlic, chilli, spices, mint and salt and pepper, then pulse until roughly chopped. Add the baking powder and egg and pulse together until well combined.

Divide and shape the chickpea mixture into golf ball-sized balls, then flatten slightly. Cover and chill in the refrigerator for 30 minutes.

Heat the oil in a large frying pan, add the falafel and cook over a medium heat for 2–3 minutes on each side until golden. Remove from the pan and drain on kitchen paper.

Meanwhile, mix all the ingredients for the dip together in a small bowl and season to taste with salt and pepper.

Serve the falafel with the mint dip, along with warmed wholemeal pitta breads.

FOR CHICKPEA FALAFEL

Place 2 x 400 g (13 oz) cans chickpeas, drained and rinsed, then drained again well, in a food processor with all the other ingredients for the falafel above, omitting the peas and using 2 tablespoons each of chopped flat leaf parsley and chopped fresh coriander in place of the mint. Continue as above.

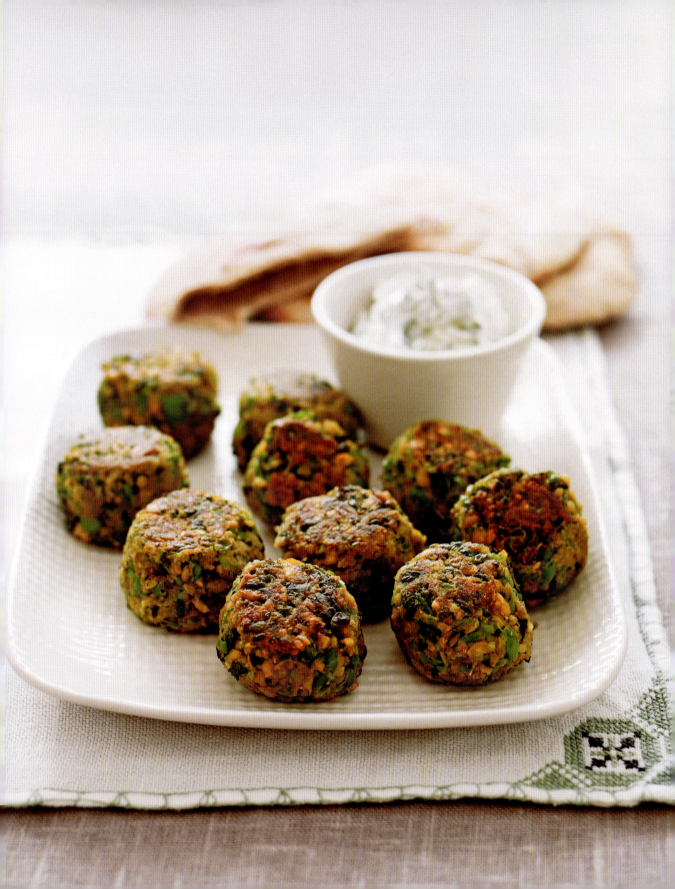

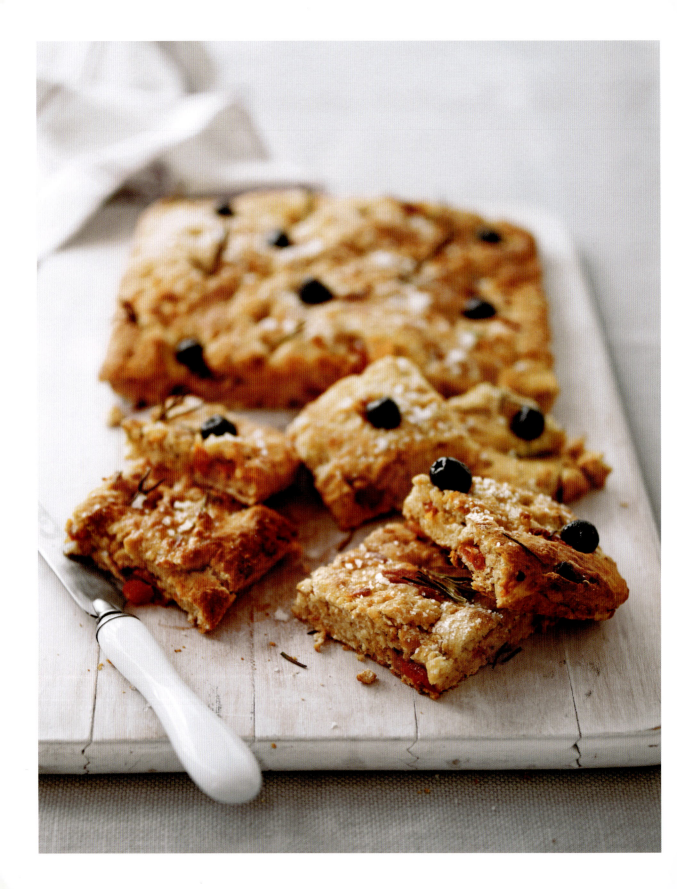

SERVES 8
PREPARATION TIME 15 MINUTES
COOKING TIME 15 MINUTES

> Homemade focaccia can be less inflammatory than store-bought because it avoids additives like emulsifiers and preservatives that may interfere with anti-inflammatory gut bacteria.

cheat's Mediterranean focaccia

olive oil, for brushing

450 g (14½ oz) plain flour, plus extra for dusting

1 teaspoon bicarbonate of soda

1 teaspoon salt

1 tablespoon chopped rosemary, plus 10 small sprigs

100 g (3½ oz) sun-dried tomatoes, chopped

400 ml (14 fl oz) buttermilk

10 pitted black olives

1 teaspoon sea salt

Brush a 32 x 23 cm (12½ x 9 inch) Swiss roll tin generously with oil.

Sift the flour, bicarbonate of soda and salt into a large bowl. Stir in the chopped rosemary and sun-dried tomatoes. Make a well in the centre, add the buttermilk to the well and gradually stir into the flour. Bring the mixture together with your hands to form a soft, slightly sticky dough.

Tip the dough out on to a lightly floured surface and lightly knead for 1 minute, then quickly roll into a rectangular shape to fit the prepared tin. Press the dough gently into the tin, then brush with oil. Using your finger, make small dimples in the top of the bread. Scatter over the black olives, rosemary sprigs and sea salt.

Bake in a preheated oven, 220°C (425°F), Gas Mark 7, for 15 minutes until brown and crisp. Brush with a little more olive oil and serve warm.

SERVES 4

PREPARATION TIME 5 MINUTES

harissa & tahini hummus

400 g (13 oz) can chickpeas, drained and rinsed

1 tablespoon tahini paste

1 garlic clove, peeled

4 tablespoons Greek yogurt

1 tablespoon rose harissa paste, plus extra for drizzling

2 tablespoons lemon juice

salt and pepper

warmed flatbreads, to serve

Place all the ingredients in a food processor, reserving a few chickpeas for garnish, and blend to a smooth paste. If the consistency is too thick, add a little warm water.

Season to taste, transfer to a serving bowl and garnish with the reserved chickpeas and a drizzle of extra harissa. Serve with warmed flatbreads.

FOR MOROCCAN PAN-ROASTED CHICKPEAS

Drain a 400 g (13 oz) can chickpeas and dry on kitchen paper. Place in a bowl and sprinkle over 2 tablespoons Moroccan spice mix, such as ras el hanout, and stir well to coat. Heat 2 tablespoons olive oil in a large frying pan and cook the chickpeas for 5–6 minutes, stirring occasionally, until golden. Transfer to a bowl and serve hot or cold.

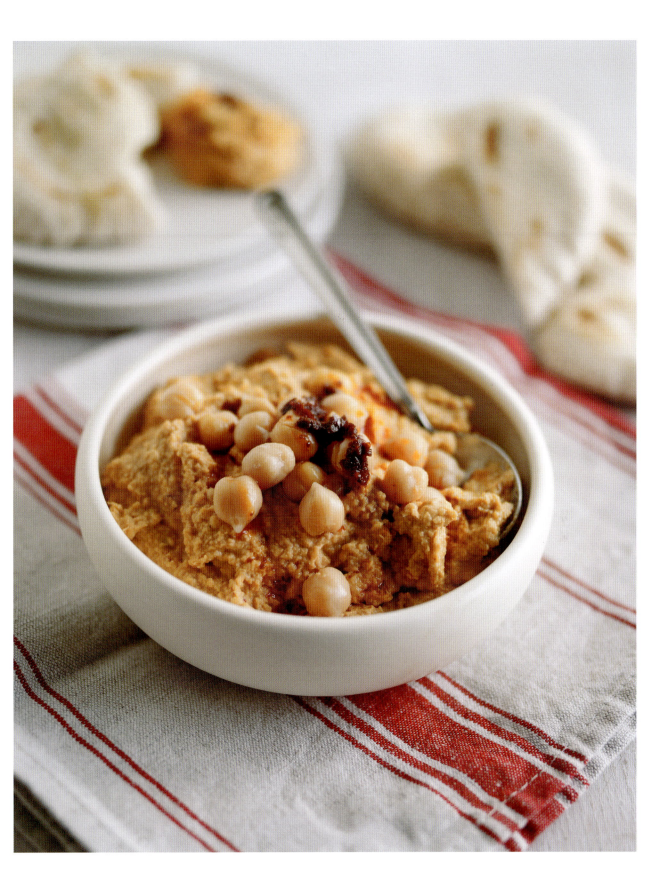

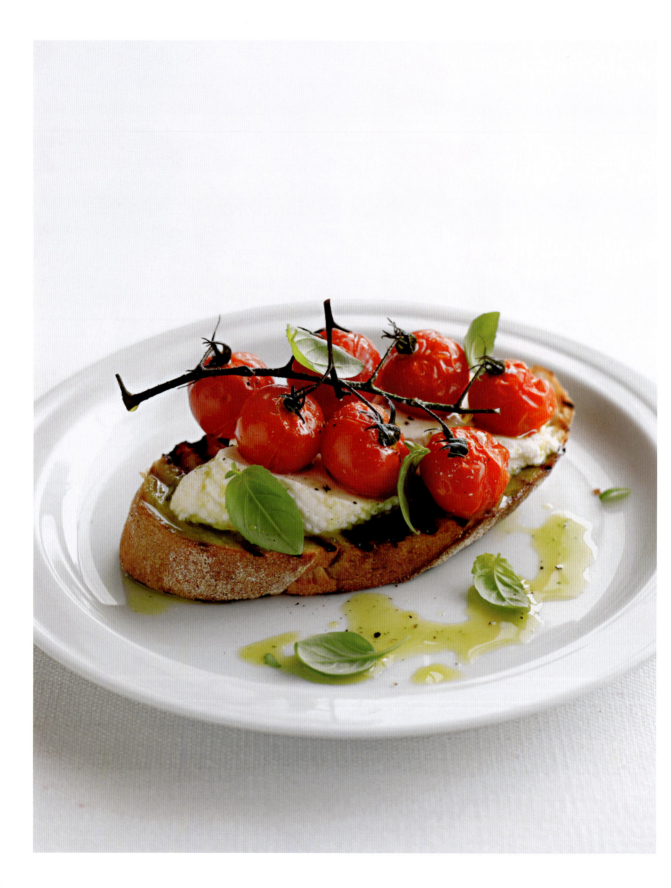

SERVES 4

PREPARATION TIME 10 MINUTES

COOKING TIME 15 MINUTES

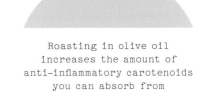

Roasting in olive oil increases the amount of anti-inflammatory carotenoids you can absorb from fresh tomatoes.

bruschetta with tomatoes & ricotta

500 g (1 lb) vine-ripened cherry tomatoes

2 tablespoons extra virgin olive oil

4 large slices of sourdough bread

1 large garlic clove, peeled

350 g (11½ oz) ricotta cheese

½ quantity Basil Oil

salt and pepper

basil leaves, to garnish

BASIL OIL

25 g (1 oz) basil leaves

150 ml (¼ pint) extra virgin olive oil

Spread the tomatoes out in a roasting tin, season with salt and pepper and drizzle with the extra virgin olive oil. Roast in a preheated oven, 220°C (425°F), Gas Mark 7, for 15 minutes.

Meanwhile, heat a ridged griddle pan until hot. Add the bread slices and cook until toasted and charred on both sides. Rub all over with the peeled garlic clove.

Make the basil oil. Plunge the basil leaves into a saucepan of boiling water, return to the boil and boil for 30 seconds. Drain the basil, refresh under cold water and dry thoroughly with kitchen paper. Transfer the oil and basil leaves to a blender and blend until really smooth.

Top each bruschetta with a slice of ricotta and the roasted tomatoes, and drizzle over the basil oil. Garnish with basil leaves.

FOR BRUSCHETTA WITH FIG, ROCKET & FETA

Toast 4 slices of sourdough bread as in the recipe above and rub each slice with garlic. Combine 4 quartered fresh figs with 150 g (5 oz) crumbled feta cheese, a good handful of baby rocket leaves and some chopped mint. Arrange on the bruschetta and serve drizzled with extra virgin olive oil.

SERVES 4

PREPARATION TIME 10 MINUTES

COOKING TIME 20 MINUTES

parsnip & beetroot crisps with homemade dukkah

rapeseed or groundnut oil, for deep-frying

2 parsnips, peeled, halved and thinly sliced lengthways

2–3 raw beetroot, peeled and thinly sliced

salt and pepper

FOR THE SPICE MIX

1 tablespoon hazelnuts

1 tablespoon sesame seeds

2 teaspoons cumin seeds

2 teaspoons coriander seeds

2 teaspoons dried mint

To make the spice mix, dry-fry the hazelnuts and seeds in a small, heavy-based frying pan over a medium heat for 2–3 minutes until they emit a nutty aroma. Using a pestle and mortar, pound the nuts and seeds to a coarse powder, or tip into a spice grinder and grind to a fine powder. Stir in the dried mint and season well. Set aside.

In a deep saucepan, heat enough oil for deep-frying to 180–190°C (350–375°F), or until a cube of bread browns in 30 seconds. Deep-fry the parsnips in batches until lightly golden. Remove with a slotted spoon and drain on kitchen paper, then tip all the parsnips into a bowl while hot and sprinkle over half the dukkah spice mix.

Reduce the heat (the beetroot slices burn easily) and deep-fry the beetroot in batches. Remove and drain as above, then tip into a bowl and sprinkle with the remaining spice mix. Serve the parsnip and beetroot crisps separately, or mixed together.

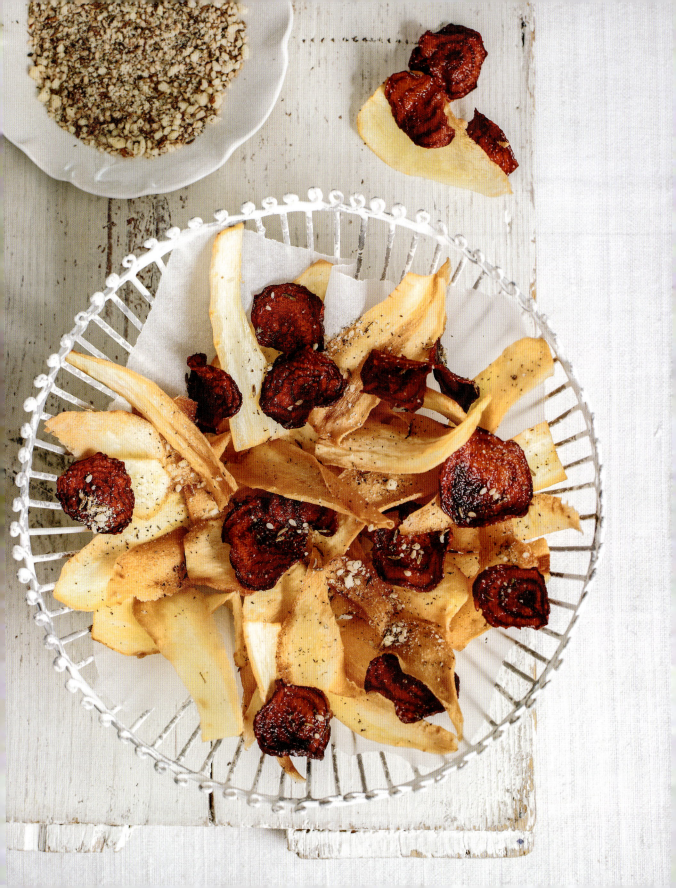

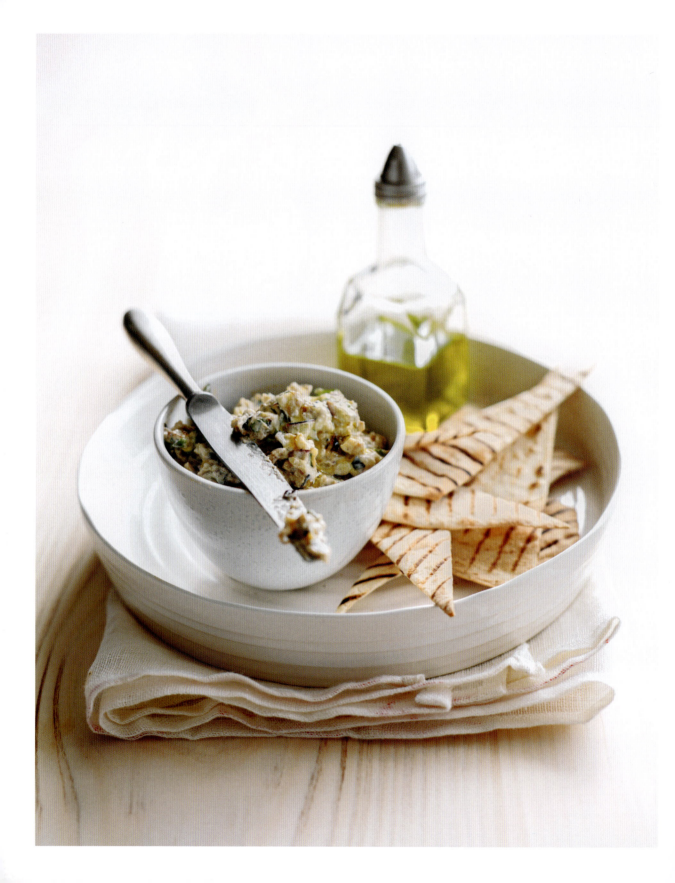

SERVES 6
PREPARATION TIME 15 MINUTES, PLUS COOLING
COOKING TIME 15 MINUTES

aubergine dip with flatbreads

1 large aubergine

4 tablespoons extra virgin olive oil

1 teaspoon ground cumin

150 ml (¼ pint) Greek-style yogurt

1 small garlic clove, crushed

2 tablespoons chopped fresh coriander

1 tablespoon lemon juice

4 flour tortillas

salt and pepper

Cut the aubergine lengthways into 5 mm (¼ inch) thick slices. Mix 3 tablespoons of the oil with the cumin and salt and pepper and brush all over the aubergine slices. Cook in a preheated ridged griddle pan or under a preheated hot grill for 3–4 minutes on each side until charred and tender. Leave to cool, then finely chop.

Mix the aubergine into the yogurt in a bowl, then stir in the garlic, coriander, lemon juice, the remaining oil and salt and pepper to taste. Transfer to a serving bowl.

Cook the tortillas in the preheated griddle pan or under the preheated hot grill for 3 minutes on each side until toasted. Cut into triangles and serve immediately with the aubergine dip.

FOR CUCUMBER & MINT DIP

Finely grate ½ cucumber and squeeze dry, then put in a bowl and stir in the remaining dip ingredients as above, replacing the coriander with an equal amount of chopped mint.

SERVES 2
PREPARATION TIME 1 MINUTE
COOKING TIME 8–9 MINUTES

'Meaty' portobello mushrooms are rich in selenium, an antioxidant that helps with immune function.

ricotta-stuffed mushrooms

4 large flat chestnut or portobello mushrooms

2 tablespoons garlic-infused olive oil

salt and pepper

rocket salad, to serve

FILLING

200 g (7 oz) ricotta cheese

12 large basil leaves, roughly chopped

finely grated rind of 1 lemon

25 g (1 oz) Parmesan cheese, grated

25 g (1 oz) pine nuts

Remove the stalks from the mushrooms and brush all over with the oil. Season to taste and place on a baking sheet, skin side up. Cook under a preheated hot grill for 5 minutes.

Meanwhile, mix all the filling ingredients in a bowl and season to taste. Turn the mushrooms over and pile the filling into the cavities, pressing it down.

Cook for a further 3–4 minutes until the filling is golden and the mushrooms are cooked through. Serve immediately with a rocket salad.

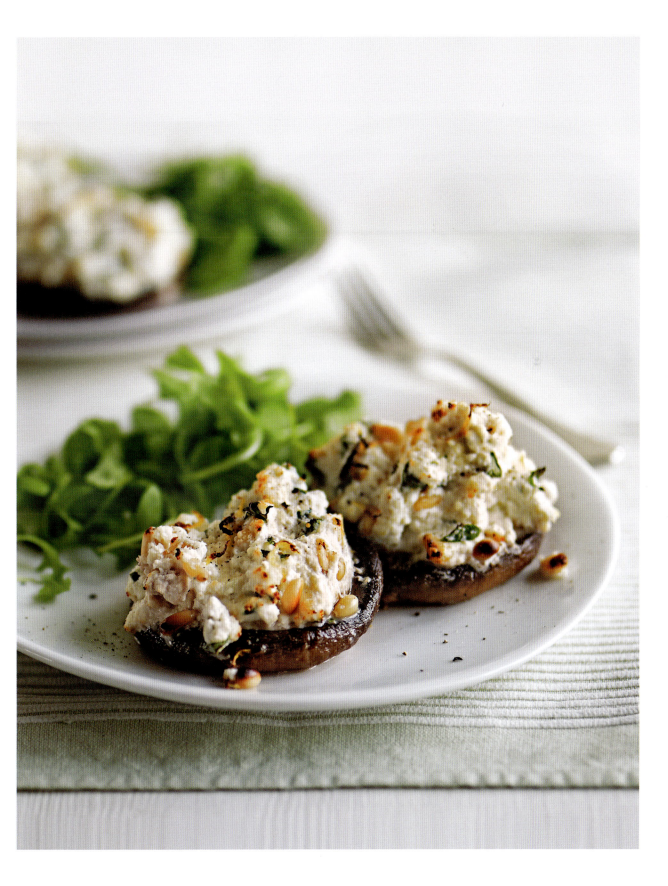

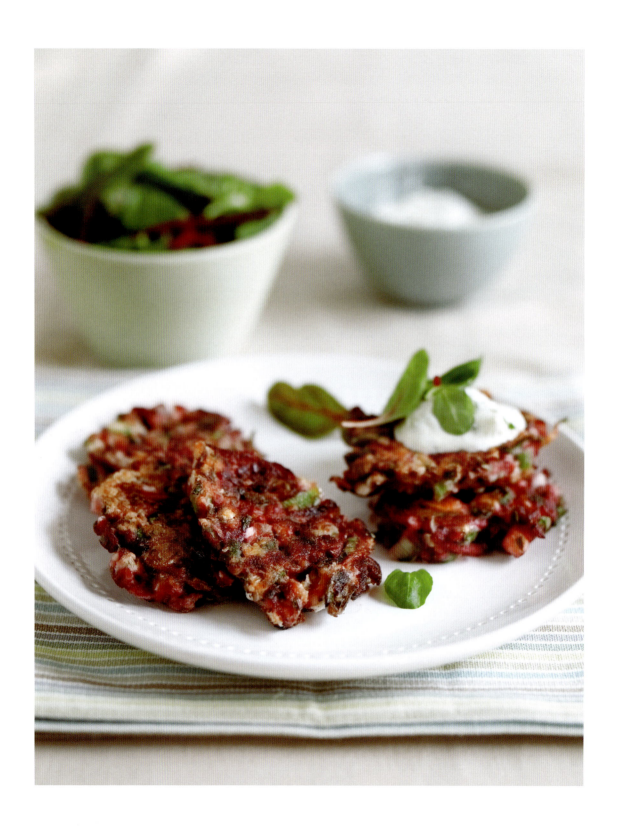

SERVES 4

PREPARATION TIME 10 MINUTES

COOKING TIME 6–12 MINUTES

courgette, beetroot & feta fritters

1 large courgette, grated

grated rind of 1 lemon

2 spring onions, sliced

2 tablespoons chopped parsley

2 tablespoons chopped mint

100 g (3½ oz) feta cheese, crumbled

2 tablespoons rice flour

1 egg yolk

2 cooked beetroot, peeled and grated

2 tablespoons olive oil

salt and pepper

basil leaves, to garnish

mixed leaf salad, to serve

Mix together the courgette, lemon rind, spring onions, herbs, feta, rice flour and egg yolk in a large bowl and season well. Gently stir in the beetroot until the mixture is just speckled with red.

Heat a little of the oil in a frying pan, add tablespoons of the mixture to the pan and fry the fritters for 1–2 minutes on each side until golden. Transfer to a serving plate and keep warm while frying the remaining mixture, adding the remaining oil to the pan as necessary.

Garnish the fritters with basil leaves and serve with a mixed leaf salad.

FOR CUCUMBER & YOGURT DIP, TO SERVE AS AN ACCOMPANIMENT

Mix together 200 ml (7 fl oz) Greek yogurt, 1 crushed garlic clove, 1 teaspoon toasted cumin seeds, ¼ grated cucumber, squeezed of excess liquid, and a pinch of paprika in a serving dish. Season well.

SERVES 6–8

PREPARATION TIME 25 MINUTES

COOKING TIME 10–12 MINUTES

chicken bites with salsa

300 g (10 oz) masa harina or fine cornmeal

½ teaspoon salt

300 ml (½ pint) hot water

4–6 tablespoons vegetable oil

plain flour, for dusting

1 cooked chicken breast, shredded

SALSA

1 green chilli, deseeded (optional) and chopped

1 garlic clove, chopped

3 canned tomatillos or 1 large tomato

2 spring onions, chopped

handful of fresh coriander leaves, chopped

Place the masa harina or cornmeal in a bowl and add the salt. Add the measured water and 2 tablespoons of the oil and mix together to form a dough. Divide the dough into 16 equal pieces and roll each into a ball, then roll out on a lightly floured work surface into 5 cm (2 inch) diameter rounds. Alternatively, flatten the dough pieces using a tortilla press. Heat a large, dry nonstick frying pan until hot, add the half the tortillas and cook for 1–2 minutes on each side until just golden and a little charred. Repeat with the remaining tortillas.

Meanwhile, make the salsa. Place all the ingredients in a food processor or blender and whizz to form a coarse purée.

Heat 2 tablespoons of the oil in a frying pan, add half the tortillas and cook for about 2 minutes on each side until golden. Remove from the pan and set aside. Repeat with the remaining tortillas, adding more oil if needed.

Arrange the crispy tortillas on a serving plate, scatter over the chicken and drizzle over the salsa. Serve immediately.

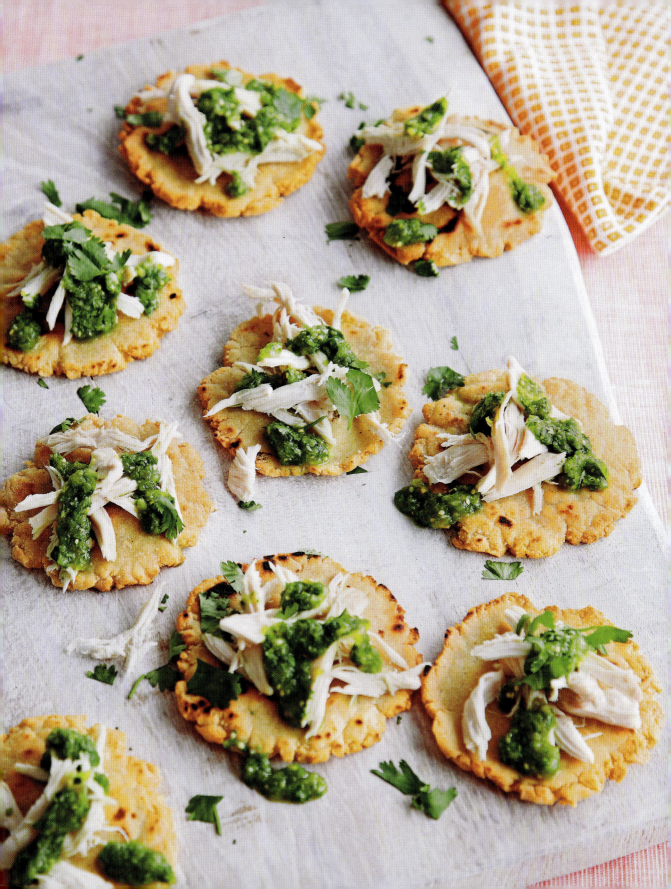

SERVES 4–6

PREPARATION TIME 10 MINUTES, PLUS COOLING

COOKING TIME 10 MINUTES

Rosemary, like many herbs, has potent antioxidant and anti-inflammatory properties, so be liberal with your sprinkle.

bean, lemon & rosemary hummus

6 tablespoons extra virgin olive oil, plus extra to serve

4 shallots, finely chopped

2 large garlic cloves, crushed

1 teaspoon chopped rosemary, plus extra sprigs to garnish

grated rind and juice of ½ lemon

2 × 400 g (13 oz) cans butter beans

salt and pepper

toasted ciabatta, to serve

Heat the oil in a frying pan, add the shallots, garlic, chopped rosemary and lemon rind and cook over a low heat, stirring occasionally, for 10 minutes until the shallots are softened. Leave to cool.

Transfer the shallot mixture to a food processor, add all the remaining ingredients and process until smooth.

Spread the hummus on to toasted ciabatta, garnish with rosemary sprigs and serve drizzled with oil.

FOR CHICKPEA & CHILLI HUMMUS

Put 2 × 400 g (13 oz) cans drained chickpeas in a food processor with 2 deseeded and chopped red chillies, 1 large crushed garlic clove, 2 tablespoons lemon juice and salt and pepper to taste. Process with enough extra virgin olive oil to form a soft paste. Serve as a dip with vegetable crudités.

SERVES 4

PREPARATION TIME 10 MINUTES

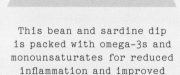

This bean and sardine dip is packed with omega-3s and monounsaturates for reduced inflammation and improved heart health.

smashed bean & sardine dip

400 g (13 oz) can cannellini beans, rinsed and drained

400 g (13 oz) can chickpeas, rinsed and drained

2 garlic cloves, crushed

juice of 1 lime

1 teaspoon ground cumin

75 g (3 oz) canned sardines, drained

100 ml (3½ fl oz) thick natural yogurt

1 tablespoon chopped fresh coriander

1 tablespoon olive oil

salt and pepper

vegetable crudités, to serve

Place the beans and chickpeas, reserving 1 tablespoon of each, in a food processor. Add the garlic, lime juice, cumin, sardines and yogurt and process until smooth.

Stir in the reserved beans and chickpeas with the coriander and season to taste. Transfer to a bowl and pour over the oil.

Serve the dip with vegetable crudités.

SERVES 4

PREPARATION TIME 10 MINUTES

COOKING TIME 20 MINUTES

These kebabs provide two of your five-a-day, plus calcium and protein from the yogurt dip.

vegetable kebabs with harissa yogurt

1 aubergine, cut into chunks

2 courgettes, cut into chunks

2 peppers, deseeded and cubed

2 onions, cut into chunks

8–12 cherry tomatoes

2 tablespoons olive oil

juice of 1 lemon

2 garlic cloves, crushed

1 teaspoon ground coriander

1 teaspoon ground cinnamon

2 teaspoons runny honey

salt and pepper

FOR THE YOGURT

400 ml (14 fl oz) natural yogurt

2 garlic cloves, crushed

2–3 teaspoons harissa paste

1 small bunch of coriander, chopped

1 small bunch of mint, chopped

Place all the vegetables and tomatoes in a non-metallic bowl. Mix together the oil, lemon juice, garlic, ground spices and honey in a small bowl, then season and pour over the vegetables. Toss well and leave to marinate for 5 minutes.

To make the harissa yogurt, mix together the yogurt, garlic and harissa in a separate bowl, season and stir in the herbs, reserving some for garnish.

Using your hands, toss the vegetables and tomatoes gently in the marinade, then thread alternately on to 8 metal skewers. Cook over a barbecue or under a preheated grill, brushing with any remaining marinade, for 3–4 minutes on each side until browned and tender. Sprinkle with the reserved herbs and serve immediately with the harissa yogurt.

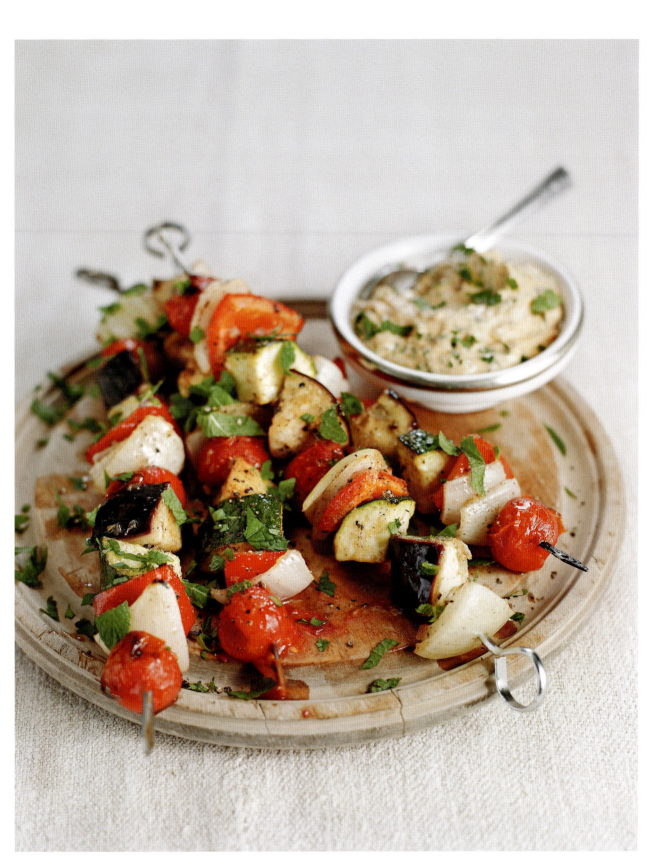

Main Meals to Heal

122	**asparagus, mint & lemon risotto**
125	**roasted salmon & vegetables**
126	**spiced tofu, noodles & pak choi**
128	**chargrilled chicken with salsa & fruity couscous**
129	**lemony prawns & broccoli stir-fry**
130	**Mediterranean-style vegetable pie**
133	**creamy paprika chicken**
134	**spiced mackerel fillets**
137	**vegetable spaghetti Bolognese**
138	**roasted butternut squash risotto**
141	**turkey balls with minty quinoa**
142	**chicken, lemon & olive stew**
144	**veggie kebabs with bulgar wheat**
145	**garlic & tomato seafood spaghetti**
146	**vegetable 'paella' with almonds**
149	**crusted salmon with tomato salsa**
150	**aubergine bake**
153	**spicy Mediterranean pasta**
154	**spinach & fish pie**
157	**Mediterranean olive chicken**

SERVES 4
PREPARATION TIME 10 MINUTES
COOKING TIME 25–30 MINUTES

asparagus, mint & lemon risotto

2 bunches of asparagus spears (about 500 g/1 lb), woody ends removed

1 vegetable stock cube

25 g (1 oz) butter

1 tablespoon olive oil

1 onion, chopped

300 g (10 oz) risotto rice

150 ml (¼ pint) dry white wine

grated rind and juice of 1 lemon

4 tablespoons chopped mint

50 g (2 oz) Parmesan cheese, grated, plus extra to serve

Chop the asparagus stalks finely, leaving the tips whole. Cook the tips and stalks in a saucepan of simmering water for about 3 minutes until al dente. Drain, reserving the cooking water.

Pour the reserved cooking water over the stock cube in a measuring jug, make up to 900 ml (1½ pints) with boiling water and stir to dissolve.

Meanwhile, melt the butter with the oil in a saucepan, add the onion and cook over a medium heat for about 2 minutes, until softened. Stir in the rice and cook for 1 minute, stirring, until well coated.

Pour in the wine and cook for 2–3 minutes until absorbed. Gradually add the hot stock, 125 ml (4 fl oz) at a time, stirring constantly and cooking until most of the liquid has been absorbed before adding the next batch of stock. Continue until almost all of the stock has been absorbed and the rice is creamy but still firm. This will take about 15 minutes.

Stir in the asparagus tips and stalks and cook for 2–3 minutes until heated through. Stir in the lemon rind and juice, mint and cheese. Cover and leave to stand for about 1 minute. Serve in bowls with extra grated cheese for sprinkling.

FOR ASPARAGUS & GOATS' CHEESE RISOTTO

Follow the recipe above to prepare the risotto, omitting the mint and cheese and stirring 125 g (4 oz) chopped creamy goats' cheese and 2 tablespoons chopped parsley into the cooked risotto. Cover and leave to stand for about 1 minute before serving.

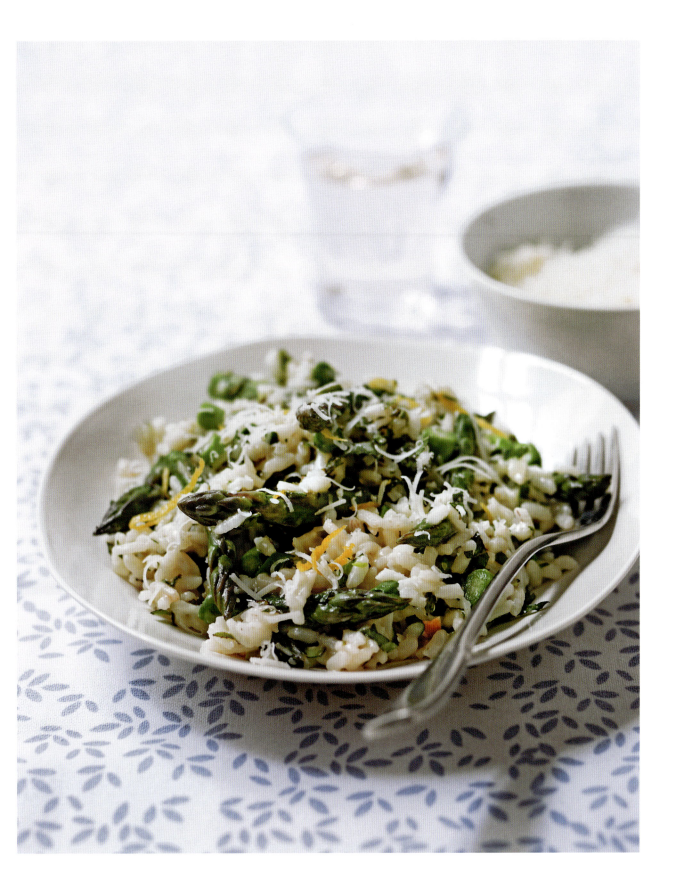

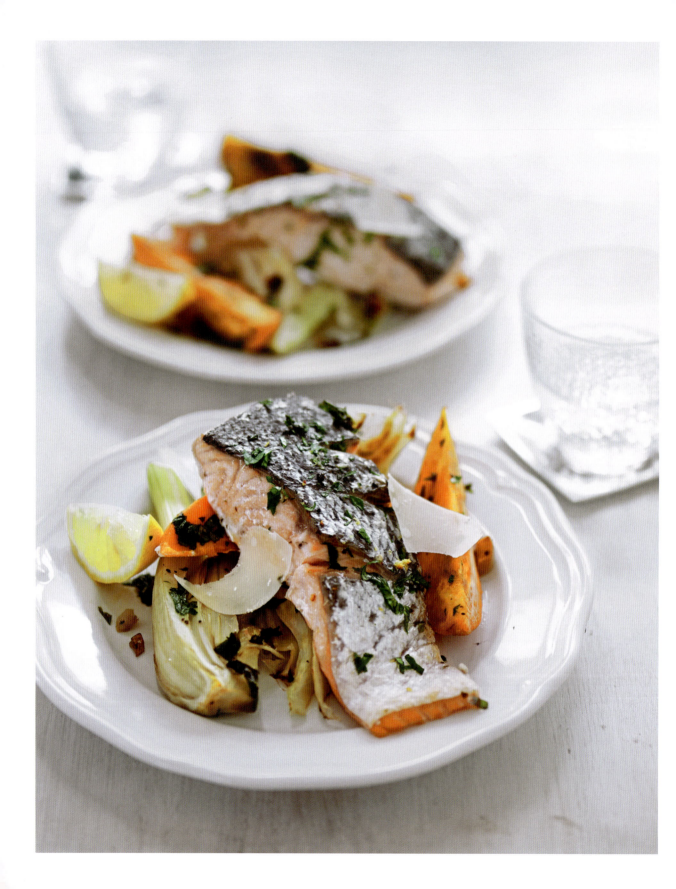

SERVES 4
PREPARATION TIME 15 MINUTES
COOKING TIME 40–45 MINUTES

> Aim for at least two portions of oily fish a week to achieve optimum intakes of the anti-inflammatory omega-3 fats EPA and DHA.

roasted salmon & vegetables

600 g (1¼ lb) sweet potatoes, peeled and cut into wedges

1 large fennel bulb, cut into 8 wedges

2 garlic cloves, chopped

1 small bunch of parsley, chopped

2 tablespoons olive oil

1 tablespoon chopped mint

4 salmon fillets, about 125 g (4 oz) each, skin scored 3 times

grated rind and juice of 1 lemon

pepper

TO SERVE

25 g (1 oz) Parmesan cheese shavings

lemon wedges

Cook the sweet potatoes and fennel in a saucepan of boiling water for 4 minutes, then drain. Transfer to a roasting tin and sprinkle with the garlic, pepper, half the parsley and the olive oil. Toss together. Roast in a preheated oven, 220°C (425°F), Gas Mark 7, for 20–25 minutes until the vegetables are tender and golden.

Meanwhile, rub the remaining parsley and the mint into the scored salmon skin. Set aside.

Lay the salmon, skin side up, on top of the vegetables, sprinkle with the lemon rind and juice and roast for a further 15 minutes, or until the fish is cooked through and the vegetables are tender.

Sprinkle with the Parmesan shavings and serve with lemon wedges.

FOR FENNEL & SALMON SOUP

Heat 1 tablespoon olive oil in a pan, add 2 chopped shallots and fry for 2–3 minutes. Add 400 g (13 oz) new potatoes and 2 chopped fennel bulbs and cook for a further 3–4 minutes. Pour in 900 ml (1½ pints) vegetable stock and simmer for 10–12 minutes until the vegetables are tender. Blend with a hand-hand blender, then return to the heat, season and drop in 400 g (13 oz) skinless salmon fillet, cut into chunks, and cook for 3–4 minutes until the fish is cooked through. Ladle into 4 bowls and serve sprinkled with chopped parsley.

SERVES 4

PREPARATION TIME 10 MINUTES, PLUS STANDING

COOKING TIME 10 MINUTES

spiced tofu, noodles & pak choi

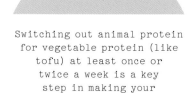

Switching out animal protein for vegetable protein (like tofu) at least once or twice a week is a key step in making your diet less inflammatory.

300 g (10 oz) firm tofu, drained

250 g (8 oz) dried medium egg noodles

1 tablespoon cornflour

½ teaspoon salt

1 teaspoon ground pepper

½ teaspoon Chinese five-spice powder

2 tablespoons sunflower oil

2.5 cm (1 inch) piece of fresh root ginger, peeled and finely chopped

1 tablespoon dark soy sauce

2 tablespoons sweet chilli sauce

100 ml (3½ fl oz) water

2 heads of pak choi, trimmed and leaves separated to the pan

Place the tofu between 2 pieces of kitchen paper and set a chopping board or other weight on top. Leave to stand for at least 10 minutes to remove excess water.

Remove the weight and kitchen paper, then cut the tofu into cubes.

Cook the noodles according to the packet instructions. Drain and set aside.

Mix together the cornflour, salt, pepper and five-spice powder in a bowl and use to coat the tofu. Heat 1 tablespoon of the oil in a wok or large frying pan over a high heat. Add the tofu and stir-fry for 2–3 minutes until golden. Remove from the pan and keep warm.

Heat the remaining oil in the pan, add the ginger and stir-fry for 1 minute. Add the noodles, stir in the soy sauce, chilli sauce and measured water, then add the pak choi. Cook, stirring, until the leaves start to wilt.

Divide the noodles between plates and top with the tofu.

FOR STIR-FRIED TOFU WITH HOISIN SAUCE

Prepare and stir-fry the tofu as above, omitting the coating. Remove from the pan and keep warm. Add 1 crushed garlic clove and 2 teaspoons chopped fresh ginger to the pan and stir-fry for 1 minute. Add 250 g (8 oz) trimmed Tenderstem broccoli, 150 g (5 oz) halved mangetout and 1 bunch of spring onions, chopped, and stir-fry for 2–3 minutes, then stir in 25 g (1 oz) toasted cashew nuts, 2 tablespoons hoisin sauce and 2 tablespoons water and 1 tablespoon soy sauce. Return the tofu to the pan and simmer for 1 minute to heat through.

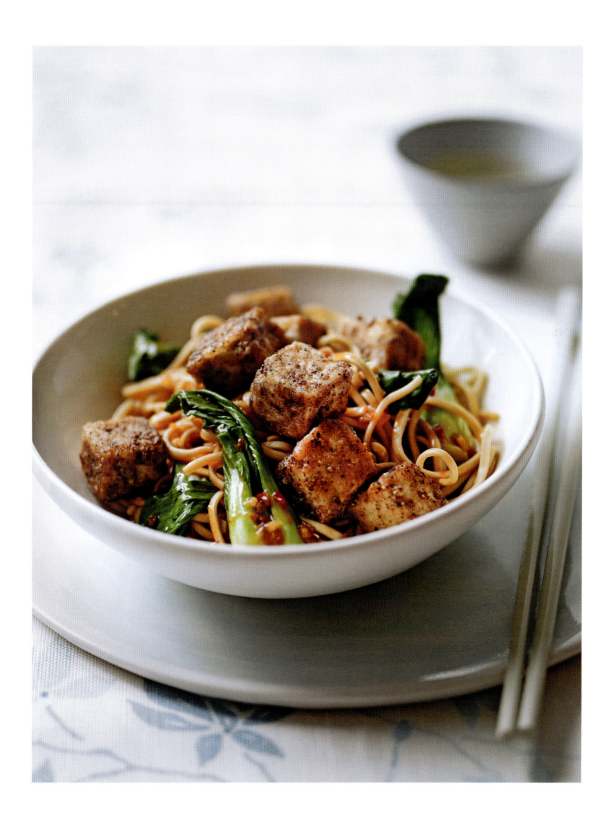

SERVES 4

PREPARATION TIME 5 MINUTES

COOKING TIME 20 MINUTES

chargrilled chicken with salsa & fruity couscous

4 boneless, skinless chicken breasts, about 150 g (5 oz) each

6 tablespoons balsamic vinegar

175 g (6 oz) wholemeal couscous

350 ml (12 fl oz) boiled water, slightly cooled

3 tablespoons olive oil

1 avocado, stoned, peeled and roughly chopped

1 large tomato, roughly chopped

5 tablespoons chopped fresh coriander

50 g (2 oz) raisins

4 tablespoons pumpkin seeds

salt

Place the chicken in a non-metallic container, pour over the vinegar and coat. Cover and leave to marinate for 5 minutes.

Place the couscous in a bowl, pour over the measured water and season with a little salt. Cover and leave to absorb the water for 10 minutes.

Meanwhile, heat 1 tablespoon of the oil in a large frying pan or griddle pan and cook the chicken over a medium heat, turning once, for 10–12 minutes until browned and cooked through.

While the chicken is cooking, make the salsa by mixing together the avocado, tomato, 1 tablespoon of the remaining olive oil and 1 tablespoon of the coriander in a bowl.

Stir the remaining tablespoon of olive oil into the couscous, then add the raisins, pumpkin seeds and remaining coriander and toss again. Serve on warmed serving plates topped with the chicken, with the salsa spooned over.

FOR SUN-DRIED TOMATO & CHICKEN COUSCOUS

Cook a 110 g (3¾ oz) pack tomato and onion couscous according to the packet instructions. Heat 3 tablespoons oil from a 185 g (6½ oz) tub sun-dried tomatoes in oil in a large saucepan and heat through 400 g (13 oz) ready-cooked chicken breast chunks for 3 minutes. Add 5 chopped sun-dried tomatoes and 1 diced red pepper and cook over a medium heat, stirring, for 5 minutes. Stir in 2 chopped spring onions, 1 tablespoon each clear honey and balsamic vinegar, 1 teaspoon wholegrain mustard and the couscous.

SERVES 4
PREPARATION TIME 5 MINUTES
COOKING TIME 30 MINUTES

lemony prawns & broccoli stir-fry

175 g (6 oz) brown basmati rice

250 g (8 oz) tenderstem broccoli, trimmed and cut into 7 cm (3 inch) lengths

3 tablespoons vegetable oil

1 large red onion, sliced

1 bunch of spring onions, trimmed and roughly chopped

250 g (8 oz) cooked peeled prawns

finely grated rind and juice of 1 lemon

3 tablespoons light soy sauce

salt

Bring a saucepan of lightly salted water to the boil and cook the rice for 15–20 minutes, according to the packet instructions. Add the broccoli to the pan and cook with the rice for a further 5 minutes until both are tender. Drain well and keep warm.

Meanwhile, heat the oil in a large, heavy-based frying pan or wok and cook the onion over a medium-high heat, stirring frequently, for 5 minutes until softened. Add the spring onions and prawns and stir-fry for 4 minutes.

Add the lemon rind and juice and soy sauce to the pan and stir well, then add the drained rice and broccoli and stir-fry for 1 minute until all the ingredients are piping hot and well mixed. Serve immediately.

FOR PRAWN & BROCCOLI NOODLES

Bring a saucepan of water to the boil and cook 200 g (7 oz) medium egg noodles for 3 minutes, then drain. Trim each stem of 250 g (8 oz) tenderstem broccoli and cut lengthways into three pieces. Heat 3 tablespoons vegetable oil in a large, heavy-based frying pan or wok and stir-fry the broccoli with 1 roughly chopped bunch of spring onions, 250 g (8 oz) cooked peeled prawns and 2 small heads shredded pak choi over a medium-high heat for 4 minutes. Add the finely grated rind and juice of 1 lemon and 3 tablespoons light soy sauce and stir well. Add the drained noodles and toss until piping hot.

SERVES 4
PREPARATION TIME 30 MINUTES
COOKING TIME 1 HOUR–1 HOUR 5 MINUTES

Using red onions nets you higher amounts of quercetin, a flavonoid with strong anti-inflammatory and antioxidant effects.

Mediterranean-style vegetable pie

2 large aubergines, sliced

5 tablespoons olive oil

1 large red onion, chopped

3 garlic cloves, finely chopped

400 g (13 oz) can chopped tomatoes

125 ml (4 fl oz) red wine

1 teaspoon caster sugar

4 teaspoons finely chopped rosemary leaves

2 roasted red peppers from a jar, drained and quartered

beaten egg, to glaze

salt and pepper

FOR THE PARMESAN PASTRY

375 g (12 oz) plain flour, plus extra for dusting

175 g (6 oz) mixed butter and white vegetable fat, diced

50 g (2 oz) Parmesan cheese, grated, plus extra for sprinkling

2 tablespoons finely chopped rosemary leaves, plus extra for sprinkling

4–4½ tablespoons cold water

Arrange the sliced aubergines on a foil-lined grill rack, drizzle with 2 tablespoons oil and sprinkle with salt and pepper. Grill for 5 minutes until browned, turn over, oil and season again, grill for a further 5 minutes, then set aside.

Heat the remaining oil in a saucepan, add the onion and fry for 5 minutes until softened. Add the garlic, tomatoes, wine, sugar and rosemary, then season well with salt and pepper. Simmer, uncovered, for 15 minutes, stirring from time to time until thickened, then leave to cool.

Make the pastry. Add the flour and a pinch of salt to a bowl, then rub in the fats with your fingertips or an electric mixer until you have fine crumbs. Stir in the Parmesan and rosemary, then mix in enough of the water to form a soft but not sticky dough. Knead lightly, then cut in half.

Roll one pastry half out thinly on a lightly floured board until large enough to cover a buttered 25 cm (10 inch) metal pie plate. Lift the pastry into the pie plate, then spoon one-third of the tomato sauce over the base. Arrange half the aubergines on top, cover with half the remaining sauce, then the red peppers. Repeat with the remaining aubergines and sauce.

Roll out the remaining pastry to form a lid. Brush the edge of the pastry on the plate with beaten egg. Lift the pastry lid over the pie, press the edges together and trim off any excess. Brush the top of the pie with egg, and sprinkle with rosemary and a little extra Parmesan.

Bake the pie in a preheated oven, 190°C (375°F), Gas Mark 5, for 30–35 minutes until golden. Check after 20 minutes and cover with foil if needed. Serve hot cut into wedges.

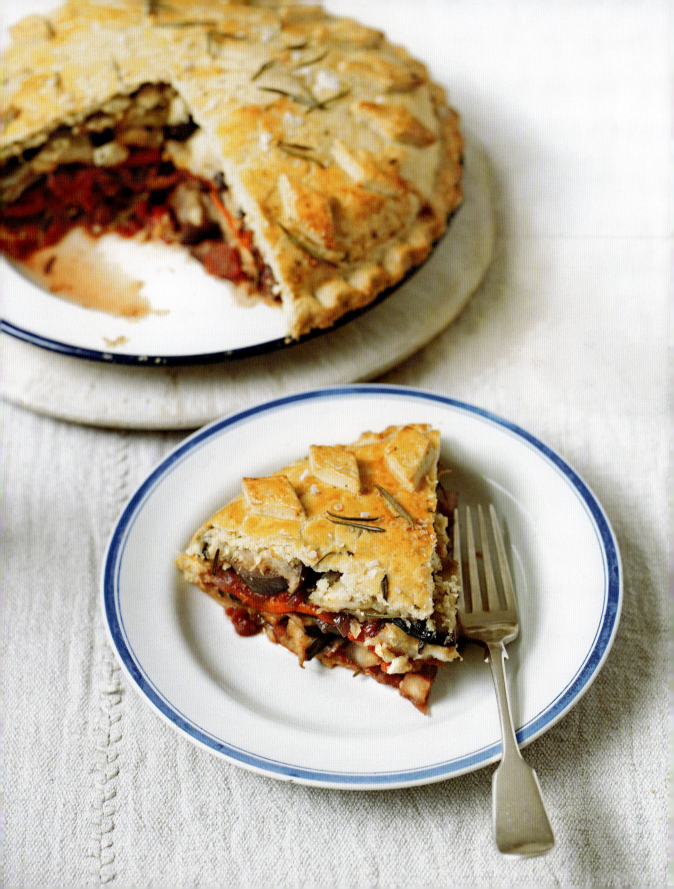

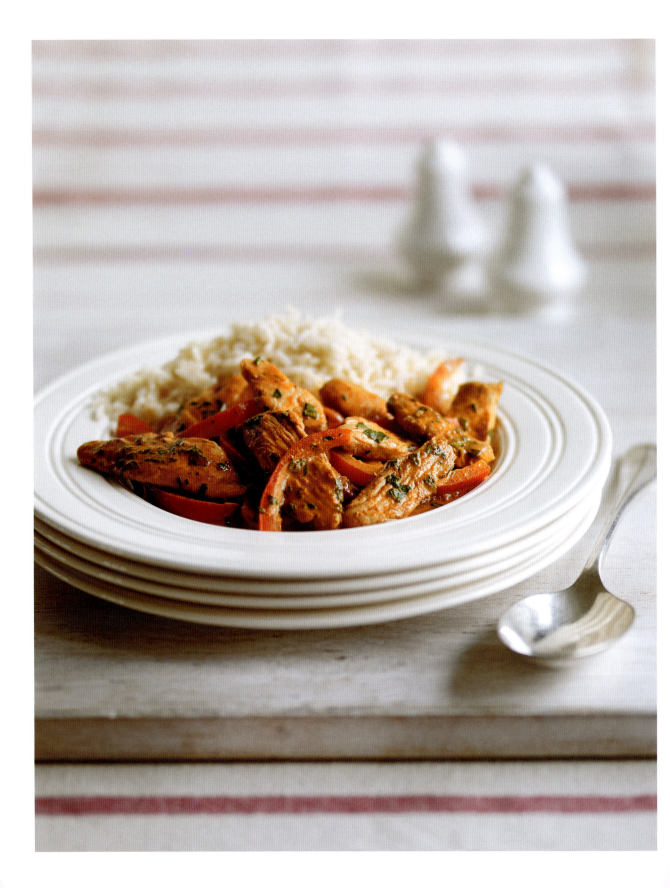

SERVES 4
PREPARATION TIME 1 MINUTE
COOKING TIME 9 MINUTES

creamy paprika chicken

15 g (½ oz) unsalted butter

1 tablespoon sunflower oil

500 g (1 lb) chicken stir-fry strips

1 red pepper, cored, deseeded and sliced

2 tablespoons sweet paprika

100 ml (3½ fl oz) medium dry sherry

2 teaspoons tomato purée

4 tablespoons crème fraîche or soured cream

1 tablespoon chopped parsley

salt and pepper

cooked rice, to serve

Heat the butter and oil in a large frying pan and stir-fry the chicken strips for 3 minutes over a high heat, until lightly browned.

Add the sliced red pepper and paprika and cook for 2 minutes, then add the sherry and tomato purée, bring to the boil and simmer for 2–3 minutes.

Stir in the crème fraîche and parsley, season to taste and heat through. Serve with rice.

FOR CREAMY PESTO CHICKEN WITH LEMON

Cook 500 g (1 lb) fresh penne in a saucepan of lightly salted boiling water according to the packet instructions. Meanwhile, heat 1 tablespoon olive oil in a frying pan with a lid, add 500 g (1 lb) chicken strips and cook for 3 minutes until lightly browned. Stir in the finely grated rind of 1 lemon, the juice of 2 lemons and 2 tablespoons fresh pesto (see page 32). Simmer for 1 minute, then stir in 3 tablespoons crème fraîche. Cover and simmer for 3–4 minutes. Drain the pasta, stir into the chicken mixture and season to taste. Serve immediately.

SERVES 4

PREPARATION TIME 4 MINUTES

COOKING TIME 5–6 MINUTES

spiced mackerel fillets

2 tablespoons olive oil

1 tablespoon smoked paprika

1 teaspoon cayenne pepper

8 mackerel fillets

2 limes, quartered

salt and pepper

rocket salad, to serve

Mix the oil with the paprika and cayenne and season to taste. Make 3 shallow cuts in the skin of each mackerel fillet and brush all over with the spiced oil.

Cook the lime quarters with the mackerel fillets on a hot barbecue or under a preheated hot grill, skin side first, for 4–5 minutes until the skin is crispy and the limes are charred.

Turn the fish over and cook for a further minute on the other side. Serve with a rocket salad.

FOR BLACK PEPPER & BAY MACKEREL

Mix together 4 very finely shredded bay leaves, 1 crushed garlic clove, ½ teaspoon freshly ground black pepper, a pinch of salt and 4 tablespoons olive oil. Rub the marinade over and into the cavities of 4 whole prepared mackerel. Cook on a hot barbecue or under a preheated hot grill for 3–4 minutes on each side. Serve alongside a tomato salad.

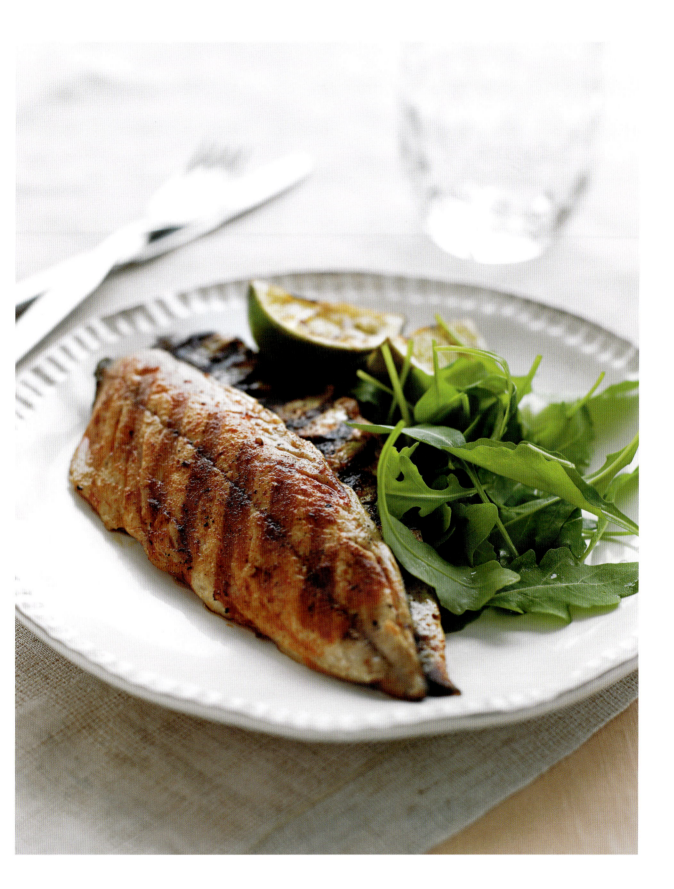

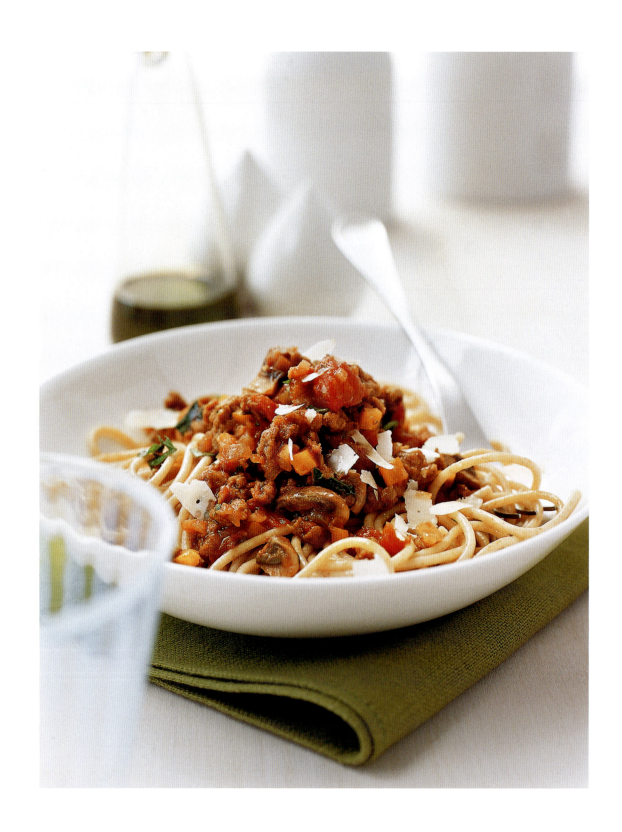

SERVES 2
PREPARATION TIME 15 MINUTES
COOKING TIME 40–50 MINUTES

> Processed tomatoes like tomato purée and canned tomatoes are a rich source of lycopene, an antioxidant that can help reduce inflammation by neutralizing free radicals and decreasing the production of pro-inflammatory substances in the body. It has been linked with improved cardiovascular health.

vegetable spaghetti Bolognese

1 tablespoon vegetable oil

1 onion, finely chopped

1 garlic clove, finely chopped

1 celery stick, finely chopped

1 carrot, finely chopped

75 g (3 oz) chestnut mushrooms, roughly chopped

1 tablespoon tomato purée

400 g (13 oz) can chopped tomatoes

250 ml (8 fl oz) red wine or vegetable stock

pinch of dried mixed herbs

1 teaspoon yeast extract

150 g (5 oz) textured vegetable protein (TVP)

2 tablespoons chopped parsley

200 g (7 oz) spaghetti

salt and pepper

grated Parmesan cheese, to serve

Heat the oil in a large heavy-based saucepan over a medium heat. Add the onion, garlic, celery, carrot and mushrooms and cook, stirring frequently, for 5 minutes or until softened. Add the tomato purée and cook, stirring, for a further minute.

Add the tomatoes, wine or stock, herbs, yeast extract and TVP. Bring to the boil, then reduce the heat, cover and simmer for 30–40 minutes until the TVP is tender. Stir in the parsley and season well.

Cook the pasta in a large saucepan of salted boiling water according to the packet instructions until it is al dente. Drain well.

Divide the pasta between 2 serving plates, top with the vegetable mixture and serve immediately with a scattering of grated Parmesan.

FOR LENTIL BOLOGNESE

Make the sauce as above, replacing the mushrooms with 1 cored, deseeded and diced red pepper and 150 g (5 oz) canned green lentils. Rinse the lentils well before use. If you are using dried lentils, cook them in boiling water first, according to the packet instructions, then drain. Cook the spaghetti as above and serve with the sauce, sprinkled with grated Parmesan cheese.

SERVES 4

PREPARATION TIME 10 MINUTES

COOKING TIME 25 MINUTES

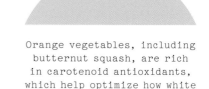

Orange vegetables, including butternut squash, are rich in carotenoid antioxidants, which help optimize how white blood cells in the immune system counter infection.

roasted butternut squash risotto

1 butternut squash, peeled, deseeded and cut into 2.5 cm (1 inch) cubes

3 tablespoons olive oil

handful of sage leaves

1 onion, chopped

200 g (7 oz) risotto rice

1 glass dry white wine

600 ml (1 pint) vegetable stock

4 tablespoons grated Parmesan cheese

15 g (½ oz) butter

75 g (3 oz) blue cheese, crumbled

75 g (3 oz) rocket leaves

salt and pepper

Put the squash on a baking sheet, drizzle over half the oil and scatter over the sage leaves. Place in a preheated oven, 200°C (400°F), Gas Mark 6, for 20–25 minutes until golden and tender.

While the squash is roasting, heat the remaining oil in a large frying pan. Add the onion and fry for 3–4 minutes until softened, then mix in the rice and coat with the oil. Pour in the wine and cook, stirring, until the liquid is absorbed.

Add the stock a ladleful at a time, stirring continually, adding the next ladle only once the previous one has been absorbed. When the rice is al dente, remove the pan from the heat, stir in the Parmesan and butter and season well.

Top the risotto with the squash and serve in shallow bowls with the blue cheese and rocket scattered over the top.

FOR WILD MUSHROOM RISOTTO

Place 15 g (½ oz) dried porcini mushrooms in a jug and pour over boiling water to just cover. Soak for 5 minutes, then chop the mushrooms and sieve the soaking liquid. Omit the squash and cook the risotto as above, adding the mushrooms and liquid with the last addition of stock. Once the rice is al dente, stir in a handful of chopped parsley and serve.

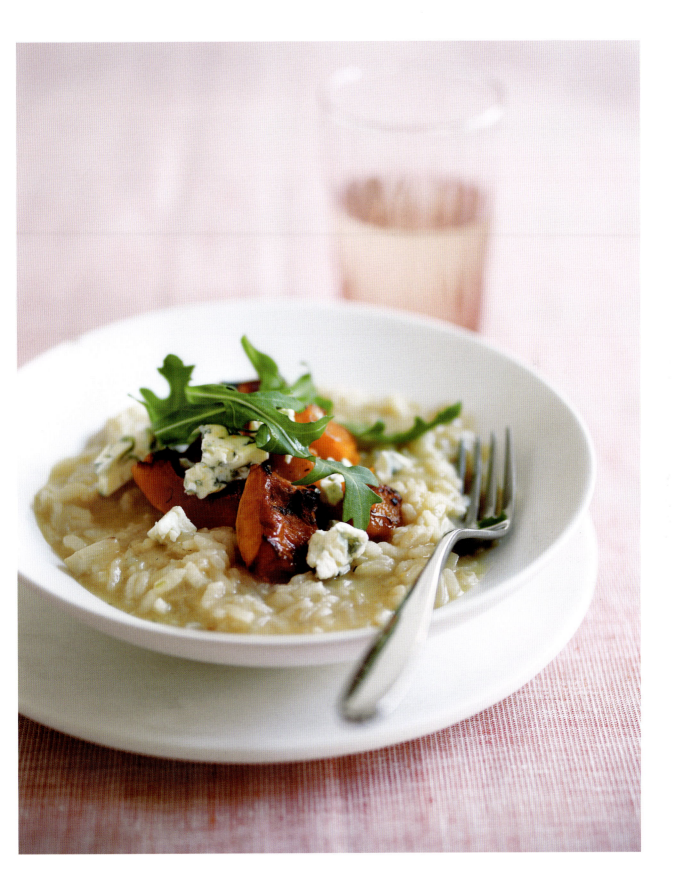

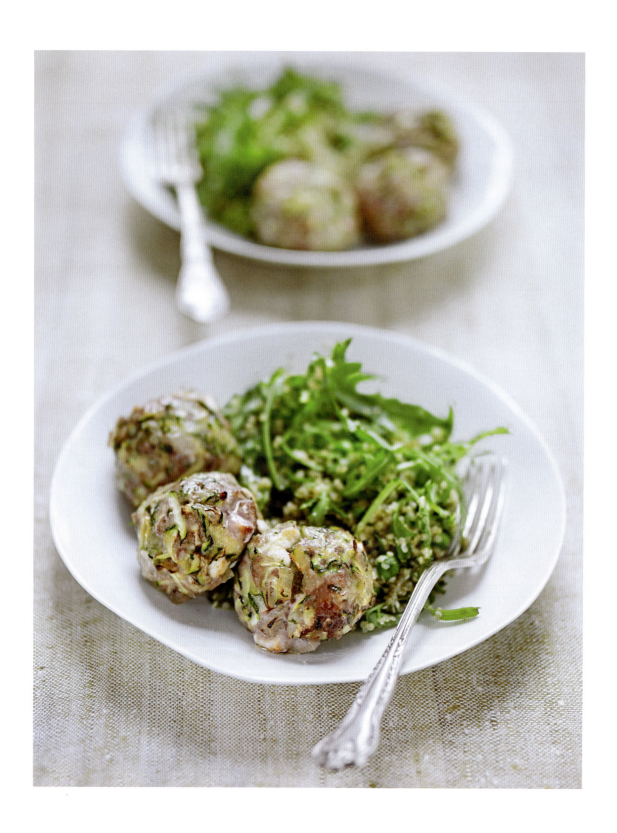

SERVES 4

PREPARATION TIME 10 MINUTES, PLUS COOLING

COOKING TIME 25 MINUTES

> Low in saturated fat, minced turkey is also a great source of vitamin B12, which helps keep the nervous system healthy.

turkey balls with minty quinoa

2 tablespoons olive oil

1 onion, finely chopped

1 garlic clove, crushed

1 courgette, grated

400 g (13 oz) minced turkey

1 teaspoon cumin seeds

50 g (2 oz) feta cheese

20 g (¾ oz) parsley, chopped

250 g (8 oz) quinoa

200 g (7 oz) frozen peas

20 g (¾ oz) mint, chopped

grated rind and juice of 1 lemon

100 g (3½ oz) rocket leaves

Heat ½ tablespoon of the oil in a frying pan, add the onion and garlic and fry for 4–5 minutes until softened. Leave to cool.

Mix together the cooked onion and garlic, courgette, turkey, cumin seeds, feta and half the parsley in a bowl. Shape into 12 balls and place on a baking sheet. Bake in a preheated oven, 200°C (400°F), Gas Mark 6, for 20 minutes until cooked through.

Meanwhile, cook the quinoa in a saucepan of boiling water according to the packet instructions. In a separate pan of boiling water, cook the peas until tender. Drain the quinoa and peas, then transfer to a bowl and stir in the mint, remaining parsley, lemon rind and juice and rocket leaves.

Serve the meatballs with the quinoa, drizzled with the remaining olive oil.

SERVES 4

PREPARATION TIME 20 MINUTES

COOKING TIME 1 HOUR

> Studies suggest curcumin — the yellow component in turmeric — can reduce inflammation, swelling and pain.

chicken, lemon & olive stew

1.5 kg (3 lb) chicken

about 4 tablespoons olive oil

12 baby onions, peeled but left whole

2 garlic cloves, crushed

1 teaspoon each ground cumin, ground ginger, ground turmeric

½ teaspoon ground cinnamon

450 ml (¾ pint) chicken stock

125 g (4 oz) kalamata olives

1 preserved lemon, pulp and skin discarded, chopped

2 tablespoons chopped fresh coriander

salt and pepper

Joint the chicken into 8 pieces (or ask your butcher to do this for you). Heat the oil in a flameproof casserole and brown the chicken on all sides. Remove the pieces with a slotted spoon and set aside.

Add the onions, garlic and spices and sauté over a low heat for 10 minutes until just golden. Return the chicken to the pan, stir in the stock and bring to the boil. Cover and simmer gently for 30 minutes.

Stir in the olives, preserved lemon and coriander and cook for a further 15–20 minutes until the chicken is really tender. Taste and adjust the seasoning, if necessary.

FOR SWEET SPINACH, TO SERVE AS AN ACCOMPANIMENT

Steam 500 g (1 lb) rinsed and drained young spinach leaves until just wilted. Drain thoroughly, then roughly chop the spinach and drain again. Heat 2 tablespoons olive oil in a pan and gently fry 1 finely chopped red onion for 2 minutes, or until translucent. Add 3 crushed garlic cloves, ¼ teaspoon chilli flakes, 50 g (2 oz) pine nuts, 50 g (2 oz) raisins and 1 teaspoon soft brown sugar (optional). Stir in the chopped spinach and cook for a further 2 minutes, until warmed through.

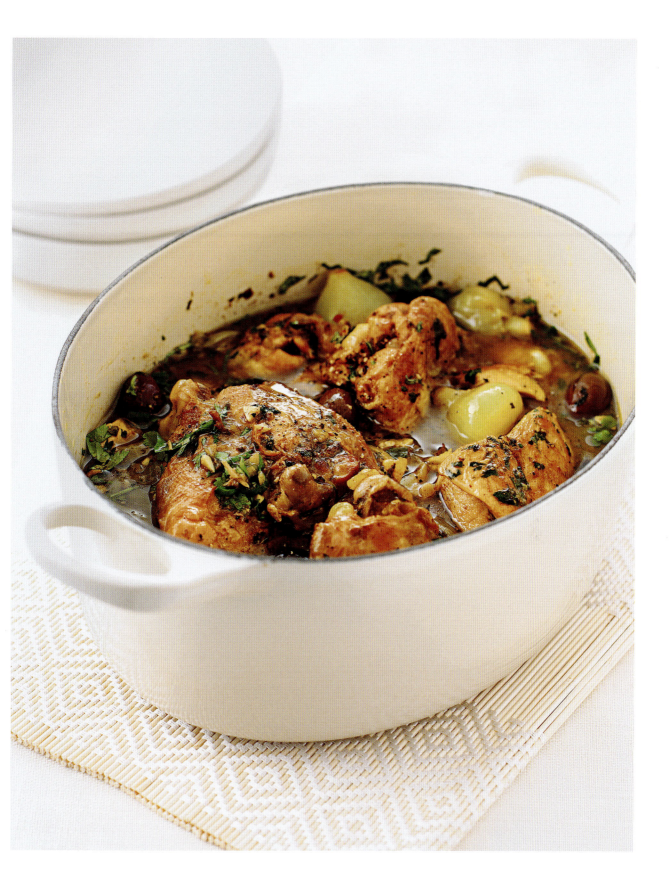

SERVES 4
PREPARATION TIME 20 MINUTES
COOKING TIME 20–25 MINUTES

> Peppers (red, yellow and green) are very rich in vitamin C — an antioxidant vitamin that helps to quell inflammation.

veggie kebabs with bulgar wheat

1 small red pepper, cored and deseeded

1 small yellow pepper, cored and deseeded

2 small courgettes, thickly sliced

1 small aubergine, cut into chunks

1 small red onion, quartered

8 chestnut mushrooms, halved

2 teaspoons dried rosemary

2 tablespoons olive oil

grated rind of 1 lemon

1 teaspoon fennel seeds

salt and pepper

BULGAR WHEAT SALAD

700 ml (23 fl oz) vegetable stock

250 g (8 oz) coarse bulgar wheat

1 tablespoon harissa paste

75 g (3 oz) raisins

2 spring onions, finely sliced

2 tablespoons chopped mint

50 g (2 oz) sunflower seeds

Cut the red and yellow peppers into large pieces and place in a bowl with the other vegetables. Toss with the dried rosemary, oil, lemon rind and fennel seeds and season with salt and pepper. Thread on to 4 long or 8 short metal skewers and cook under a medium-hot grill for 20–25 minutes, or until tender and browned, turning occasionally.

Meanwhile, put the stock in a saucepan and bring to the boil. Add the bulgar wheat, cover and simmer for 7 minutes. Remove from the heat and leave to stand until the liquid has been absorbed. Fork the harissa, raisins, spring onions, mint and sunflower seeds through the cooked bulgar wheat until well combined, then spoon on to serving plates.

Arrange the vegetable kebabs on the plates with the bulgar wheat salad and serve immediately.

FOR MINTED YOGURT, TO SERVE AS AN ACCOMPANIMENT

Mix together 250 ml (8 fl oz) fat-free Greek yogurt, ½ teaspoon fennel seeds, 2 tablespoons lemon juice and 3 tablespoons chopped mint in a serving dish and season to taste.

SERVES 4

PREPARATION TIME 10 MINUTES

COOKING TIME 25 MINUTES

garlic & tomato seafood spaghetti

225 g (7½ oz) dried wholemeal spaghetti

3 tablespoons olive oil

2 garlic cloves, sliced

3 shallots, cut into slim wedges

1 celery stick, thinly sliced

4 tomatoes, roughly chopped

400 g (13 oz) can chopped tomatoes

150 ml (¼ pint) white wine

1 tablespoon chopped thyme

3 tablespoons chopped parsley

250 g (8 oz) large cooked peeled prawns

240 g (7¾ oz) packet frozen raw mixed seafood, defrosted

salt

warm crusty bread, to serve (optional)

Bring a large saucepan of lightly salted water to the boil and cook the spaghetti for 8–10 minutes until just tender. Drain and keep warm.

Meanwhile, heat the oil in a large, heavy-based frying pan and cook the garlic, shallots and celery over a medium heat, stirring occasionally, for 3–4 minutes until slightly softened. Add the fresh tomatoes, increase the heat and cook, stirring occasionally, for 2–3 minutes. Stir in the canned tomatoes and wine.

Bring the tomato mixture to the boil, then reduce the heat slightly to a brisk simmer and cook for 8–10 minutes until the sauce has reduced by a third. Add the herbs, prawns and mixed seafood and cook for 3–4 minutes until the seafood is opaque and all is piping hot. Add the drained spaghetti and toss well to coat in the sauce.

Serve in warmed serving bowls with warm crusty bread to mop up the juices, if liked.

SERVES 4

PREPARATION TIME 25 MINUTES

COOKING TIME 30 MINUTES

Almonds contain lots of anti-inflammatory ingredients, including polyphenols, monounsaturates and vitamin E.

vegetable 'paella' with almonds

4 tablespoons olive oil

1 onion, chopped

pinch of saffron threads

225 g (7½ oz) Arborio rice

1.2 litres (2 pints) vegetable stock

175 g (6 oz) fine asparagus spears, trimmed and cut into 5 cm (2 inch) lengths

1 bunch of spring onions, cut into strips

175 g (6 oz) midi plum tomatoes on the vine, halved

125 g (4 oz) frozen peas

3 tablespoons flaked almonds, toasted

3 tablespoons chopped flat leaf parsley

salt

Heat 1 tablespoon of the oil in a large, heavy-based frying pan, add the onion and saffron and cook over a medium heat, stirring frequently, for 5 minutes, until the onion is softened and golden. Add the rice and stir well, then season with some salt. Add the stock and bring to the boil, then cover and simmer, stirring occasionally, for 20 minutes until the stock is almost all absorbed and the rice is tender and cooked through.

Meanwhile, heat the remaining oil in a separate frying pan, add the asparagus and spring onions and cook over a medium heat for 5 minutes until softened and lightly charred in places. Remove from the pan with a slotted spoon. Add the vine tomatoes to the pan and cook for 2–3 minutes on each side until softened.

Add the peas to the rice and cook for a further 2 minutes, then add the asparagus, spring onions and tomatoes and gently toss through. Scatter with the almonds and parsley and serve.

FOR PEPPER & MUSHROOM 'PAELLA' WITH PINE NUTS

Heat 2 tablespoons olive oil in a large, heavy-based frying pan, add 1 red, 1 green and 1 yellow pepper, cored, deseeded and thinly sliced, 175 g (6 oz) chestnut mushrooms, quartered, and 1 small red onion, thinly sliced, and cook over a medium heat for 4–5 minutes until softened. Add 225 g (7½ oz) Arborio rice and stir well, then season with some salt. Pour in 1.2 litres (2 pints) vegetable stock and bring to the boil, then cover and simmer for 20 minutes until the stock is almost all absorbed and the rice is tender and cooked through. Remove from the heat and stir in 3 tablespoons each lightly toasted pine nuts and chopped flat leaf parsley.

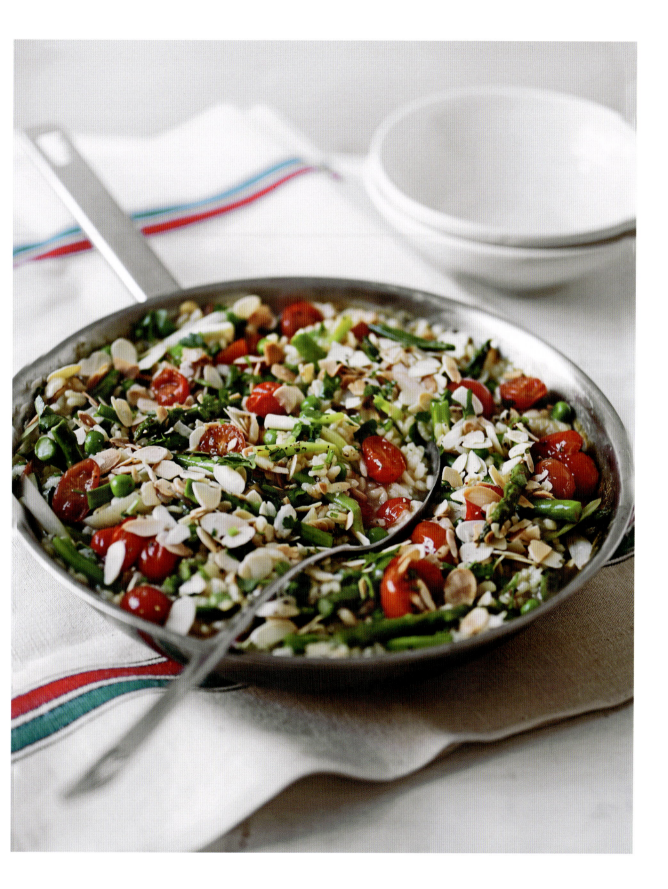

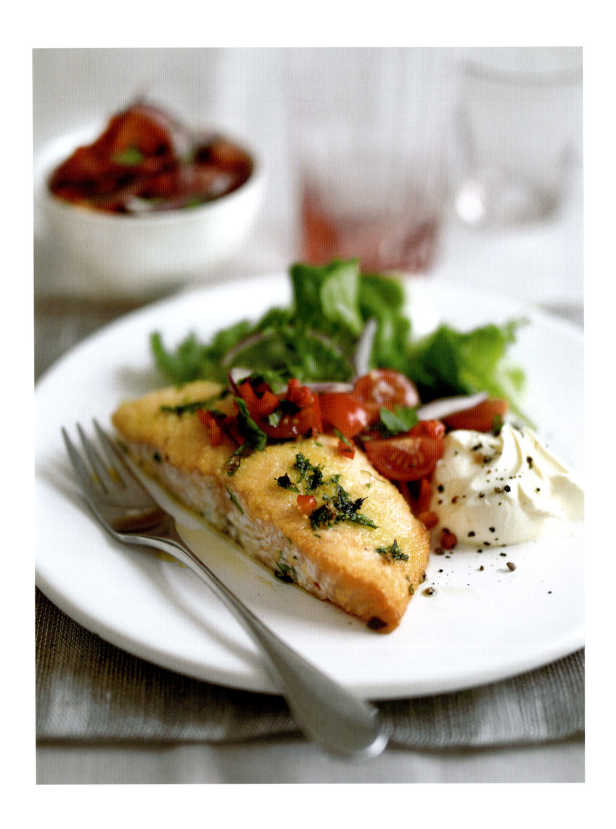

SERVES 4
PREPARATION TIME 10 MINUTES
COOKING TIME 12–15 MINUTES

crusted salmon with tomato salsa

1 tablespoon chopped fresh herbs

1 garlic clove, crushed

3 tablespoons polenta

4 pieces of skinless salmon fillet, about 125 g (4 oz) each

pepper

4 tablespoons light crème fraîche, to serve

green salad, to serve

SALSA

375 g (12 oz) cherry tomatoes, quartered

1 small red onion, finely sliced

½ red chilli, deseeded and finely chopped

handful of fresh coriander, chopped

Mix together the herbs, garlic and polenta in a shallow bowl. Coat the salmon pieces in the polenta mix, pressing it down firmly.

Put the coated fish on a baking sheet and place in a preheated oven, 200°C (400°F), Gas Mark 6, for 12–15 minutes until cooked through.

Mix together the salsa ingredients in a bowl. Place the salmon on 4 serving plates, top with the salsa and a spoonful of crème fraîche, season with pepper and serve with a green salad.

FOR POLENTA-CRUSTED CHICKEN

Beat together 2 tablespoons cream cheese with the chopped fresh herbs and 1 finely diced garlic clove. Make a horizontal slit in 4 boneless, skinless chicken breasts. Fill the cavities of the chicken breasts with the cream cheese mixture, then secure with cocktail sticks. Dip the chicken breasts in a little flour, a little beaten egg, then in the polenta. Fry in olive oil for 2–3 minutes on each side, transfer to a baking sheet and place in a preheated oven, 200°C (400°F), Gas Mark 6, for 10–12 minutes or until the chicken is cooked through. Serve with the salsa and a green salad.

SERVES 4

PREPARATION TIME 10 MINUTES

COOKING TIME 40–45 MINUTES

Mixing up your veg colours ensures you get a wider range of anti-inflammatory phytochemicals. Aubergines are a great way to get your purples!

aubergine bake

2 large aubergines, sliced

2 tablespoons olive oil

150 g (5 oz) mozzarella cheese, roughly chopped

4 tablespoons grated Parmesan cheese

salt and pepper

TOMATO SAUCE

1 tablespoon olive oil

1 garlic clove, crushed

1 small onion, finely chopped

400 g (13 oz) can plum tomatoes

handful of basil, torn

TO SERVE

salad

crusty bread

Make the tomato sauce. Heat the oil in a saucepan, add the garlic and onion and fry for 3–4 minutes until softened. Add the tomatoes and basil, bring to the boil and simmer for 15 minutes.

While the sauce is simmering, brush the aubergines with the oil on each side. Heat a griddle until hot and cook the aubergine slices for 1–2 minutes on each side until tender and browned.

Spoon a little of the tomato sauce into an ovenproof dish, layer over half the aubergines, scatter over half the mozzarella and Parmesan and season well. Repeat the layering with the remaining ingredients, finishing with a scattering of the cheeses.

Place the dish in a preheated oven, 200°C (400°F), Gas Mark 6, for 20–25 minutes until golden and bubbling. Serve with salad and crusty bread.

FOR AUBERGINE, CHILLI & CHICKEN BAKE

Make the tomato sauce as above, adding 1 deseeded and finely sliced red chilli with the garlic and onion. Cook the aubergine and layer the bake as above, interspersing 300 g (10 oz) torn cooked chicken between the aubergine layers. Bake in the oven as above.

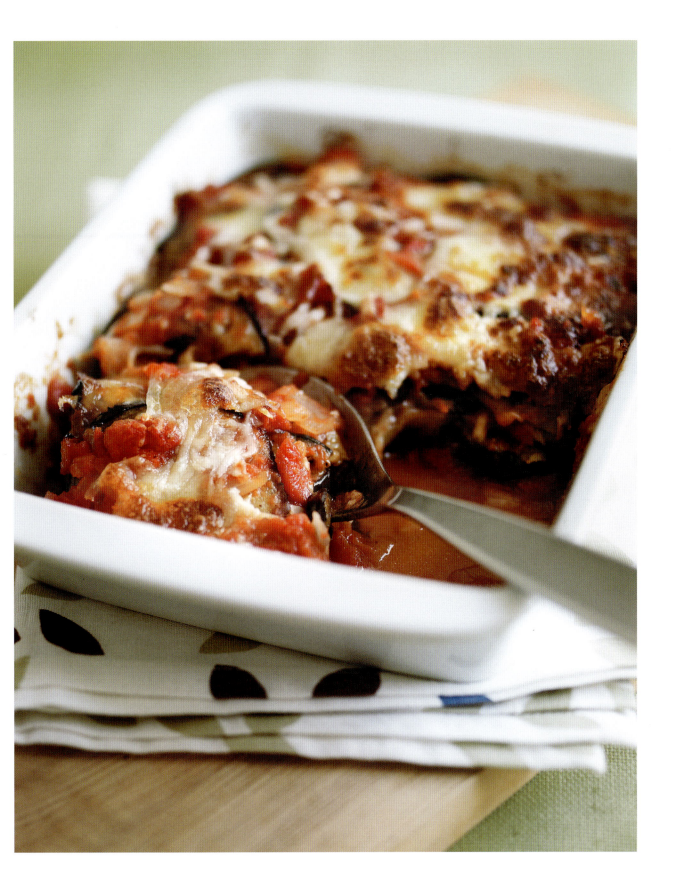

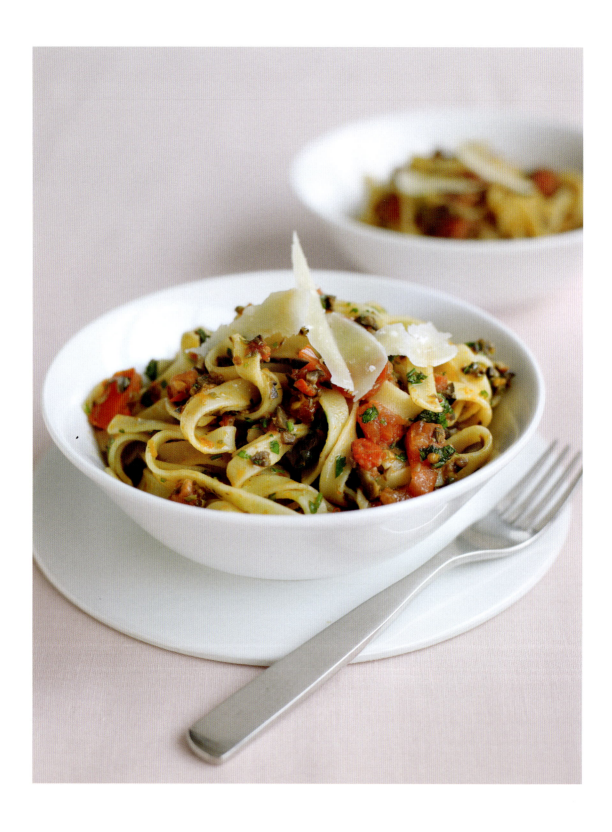

SERVES 4

PREPARATION TIME 10 MINUTES

COOKING TIME 5 MINUTES

Brown, higher-fibre grains (like wholemeal pasta) contain more anti-inflammatory components, including lignans, than their white counterparts.

spicy Mediterranean pasta

125 g (4 oz) pitted black olives

1 red chilli, deseeded and sliced

4 tablespoons capers in brine, drained

2 tablespoons sun-dried tomato paste

3 tablespoons chopped basil

3 tablespoons chopped parsley or chervil

4 tomatoes, chopped

125 ml (4 fl oz) olive oil

375 g (12 oz) wholemeal pasta shapes

salt and pepper

Parmesan cheese shavings, to serve

Place the olives, chilli and capers in a food processor or blender and process until quite finely chopped. Alternatively, finely chop them by hand. Mix with the sun-dried tomato paste, herbs, tomatoes and oil, and season to taste with salt and pepper.

Cook the pasta in plenty of lightly salted boiling water for 2–3 minutes, or according to the packet instructions, until al dente. Drain and return to the saucepan.

Add the olive mixture and toss the ingredients together lightly over a low heat for 2 minutes. Serve sprinkled with Parmesan shavings.

FOR SPICY AUBERGINE PASTA WITH PINE NUTS

Cook and drain 375 g (12 oz) pasta. Roughly chop 1 large aubergine and toss with 4 tablespoons olive oil. Roast in a preheated oven, 200°C (400°F), Gas Mark 6, for 20–25 minutes until turning golden and soft. Toss 125 g (4 oz) olives and a sliced red chilli with 2 tablespoons sun-dried tomato paste, herbs and tomato as above, but omitting the capers and remaining oil. Put in a pan with 4 tablespoons water and the aubergine and heat for 2–3 minutes. Toss with the pasta and serve in warm bowls with lightly toasted pine nuts and Parmesan cheese scattered over, and with warm crusty bread on the side.

SERVES 4
PREPARATION TIME 15 MINUTES
COOKING TIME 45–55 MINUTES

spinach & fish pie

1 tablespoon olive oil

1 onion, chopped

175 g (6 oz) baby leaf spinach

50 g (2 oz) butter

25 g (1 oz) rice flour

600 ml (1 pint) semi-skimmed milk

1 tablespoon wholegrain mustard

good grating of nutmeg

650 g (1 lb 5 oz) mixed skinless salmon, haddock and smoked haddock fillets, cut into chunks

200 g (7 oz) raw prawns, peeled and deveined

salt and pepper

POTATO TOPPING

1 kg (2 lb) potatoes, peeled and cut into chunks

good knob of butter

100 ml (3½ fl oz) single cream

Make the potato topping. Cook the potatoes in a saucepan of salted boiling water for 15 minutes or until tender. Drain well and return to the pan. Mash together with the butter and cream and season well.

Heat the oil in a large saucepan, add the onion and fry for 2–3 minutes until beginning to soften. Add the spinach to the pan and cook until wilted and any liquid has evaporated.

Melt the butter in a saucepan, add the flour and cook, stirring, for 1 minute. Gradually add the milk and cook, stirring all the time, until thickened and smooth. Stir in the mustard and nutmeg and season well.

Arrange the fish and the prawns in a large ovenproof dish. Pour the sauce over the fish, spoon the mash on top and place in a preheated oven, 200°C (400°F), Gas Mark 6, for 30–35 minutes until golden and bubbling.

FOR RÖSTI-TOPPED FISH PIE

Steam 3 peeled baking potatoes for 12–15 minutes, then grate into a large bowl. Stir in 25 g (1 oz) melted butter and season well. Make the sauce as above and pour over the fish and prawns in a large ovenproof dish. Scatter the rösti over the fish and sauce and cook as above.

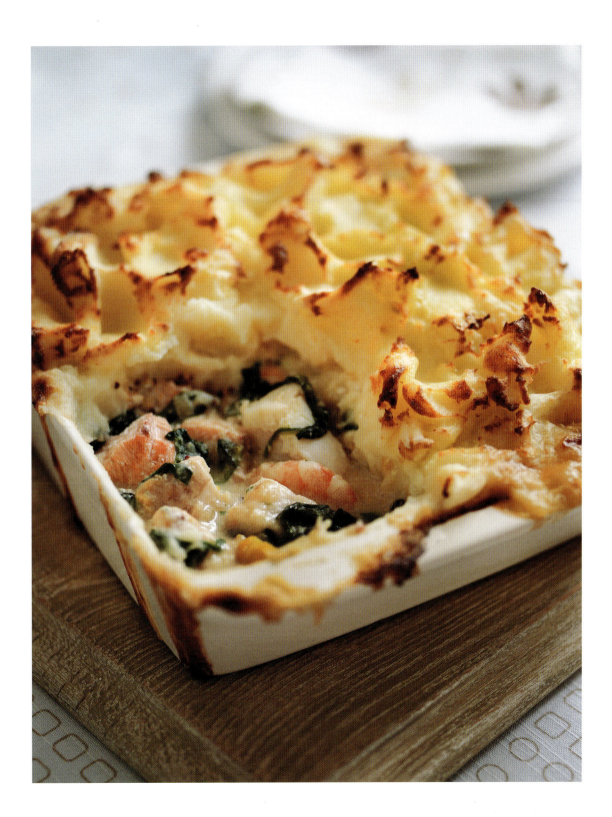

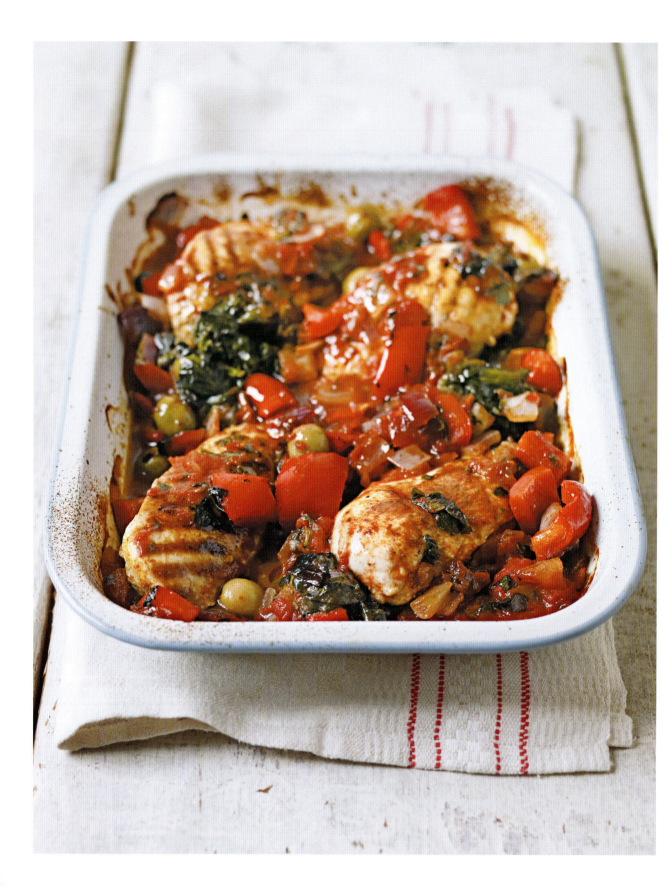

SERVES 4

PREPARATION TIME 5 MINUTES

COOKING TIME 25–30 MINUTES

Mediterranean olive chicken

4 × 150 g (5 oz) chicken breasts

½ teaspoon paprika

1 tablespoon olive oil

1 red pepper, cored, deseeded and chopped

1 red onion, chopped

1 garlic clove, crushed

400 g (13 oz) can chopped tomatoes

100 g (3½ oz) frozen spinach, defrosted

2 tablespoons green olives

1 teaspoon capers

1 tablespoon chopped basil

salt and pepper

Dust the chicken breasts with the paprika and cook on a hot griddle for 4–5 minutes on each side, then place in an ovenproof dish.

Meanwhile, heat the oil in a pan over a medium heat, add the pepper, onion and garlic and cook for 3–4 minutes. Add the chopped tomatoes, spinach, olives, capers and basil and bring to a simmer. Season to taste with salt and pepper.

Pour the sauce over the chicken and bake in a preheated oven, 200°C (400°F), Gas Mark 6, for 15–18 minutes, until the chicken is cooked through.

Light Bites & Sides

161	**veggie stir-fry with pak choi**
162	**Mediterranean-style tomato soup**
165	**sweet chilli chicken patties**
166	**butternut & cumin soup**
168	**mushroom risotto cakes**
169	**thai-style chicken soup**
170	**spiced tuna open sandwiches**
173	**honeyed pumpkin & ginger broth**
174	**ciabatta toasties with Mediterranean vegetables**
177	**tuna & jalapeño baked potatoes**
178	**mixed pickled vegetables**
180	**sweet potato & garlic mash**
181	**spiced green lentils with tomatoes**
182	**baby vegetables with pesto**
185	**broad beans with mint & lemon**
186	**roasted spiced pumpkin**
189	**asparagus with sesame dressing**
190	**sweet potatoes with green olives**

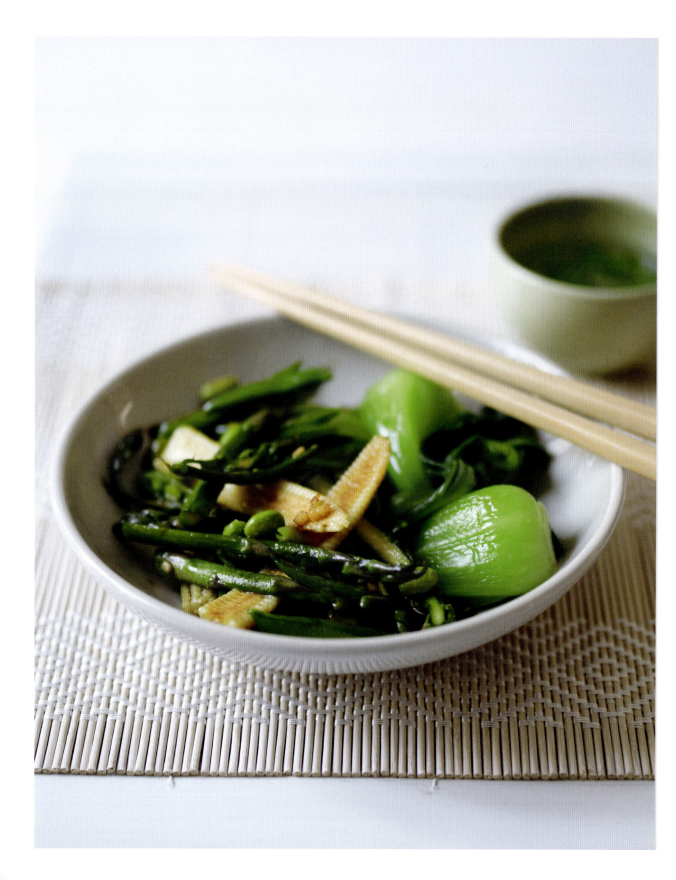

SERVES 4

PREPARATION TIME 10 MINUTES

COOKING TIME 5–7 MINUTES

> With ginger root and three of your five-a-day per serving, this veggie stir-fry has big anti-inflammatory credentials.

veggie stir-fry with pak choi

8 small pak choi, about 625 g (1¼ lb) in total

1 tablespoon groundnut oil

2 garlic cloves, thinly sliced

2.5 cm (1 inch) piece of fresh root ginger, peeled and finely chopped

200 g (7 oz) sugar snap peas, sliced diagonally

200 g (7 oz) asparagus tips, sliced in half lengthways

200 g (7 oz) baby corn, sliced in half lengthways

120 g (4 oz) podded edamame beans or 200 g (7 oz) bean sprouts

150 ml (¼ pint) sweet teriyaki sauce

steamed rice, to serve (optional)

Cut the pak choi in half, or into thick slices if large, and put in a steamer basket. Lower into a shallow saucepan of boiling water so that the pak choi is not quite touching the water. Cover and steam for 2–3 minutes or until tender. Alternatively, use a bamboo or electric steamer.

Heat a large wok or frying pan over a high heat until smoking hot, add the oil, garlic and ginger and stir-fry for 30 seconds. Add the vegetables (except the steamed pak choi) and stir continuously for 2–3 minutes or until beginning to wilt.

Pour over the sweet teriyaki sauce, toss to combine and serve immediately with the steamed pak choi and steamed rice, if liked.

FOR SWEET CHILLI VEGETABLE STIR-FRY

Heat the oil in the wok and stir-fry 1 thinly sliced onion with the garlic and ginger. Add 1 carrot, cut into thin matchsticks, and 200 g (7 oz) sliced mushrooms and stir-fry for 2 minutes. Stir in 200 g (7 oz) bean sprouts and 300 g (10 oz) shredded spinach for a further minute until wilted. Stir in 200 ml (7 fl oz) sweet chilli stir-fry sauce and serve immediately with the steamed pak choi or cooked noodles.

SERVES 2
PREPARATION TIME 5 MINUTES
COOKING TIME 20 MINUTES

Using tomatoes at their peak ripeness ensures you get the highest amount of lycopene — the antioxidant pigment that makes tomatoes red.

Mediterranean-style tomato soup

375 g (12 oz) ripe tomatoes, roughly chopped

5 tablespoons olive oil

1 garlic clove, crushed

300 ml (½ pint) hot vegetable stock

1 tablespoon tomato purée

½ teaspoon caster sugar

1 teaspoon oregano leaves, plus extra to garnish

1 tablespoon shredded basil leaves

1 ciabatta roll, torn into pieces

2 tablespoons grated Parmesan cheese

salt and pepper

Place the tomatoes in a saucepan with 2 tablespoons of the oil and the garlic. Cook for 3 minutes until softened, then add the stock, tomato purée, sugar, oregano and shredded basil. Bring to the boil, then reduce the heat, cover and simmer for 10 minutes.

Meanwhile, spread the ciabatta pieces over a baking sheet and drizzle over 2 tablespoons of the oil. Toast under a preheated medium grill for a few minutes, turning occasionally, until crisp and golden.

Blend the soup with a stick blender until smooth. Stir in half the Parmesan and season.

Ladle the soup into 2 warm serving bowls, drizzle with the remaining oil and top with some of the ciabatta croûtons. Scatter with the remaining Parmesan and a few oregano leaves. Serve topped with the remaining ciabatta croûtons.

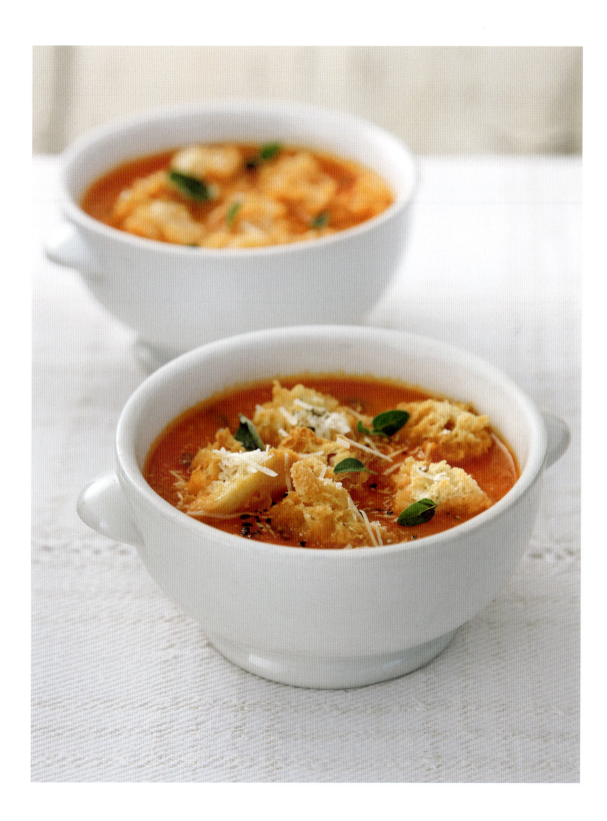

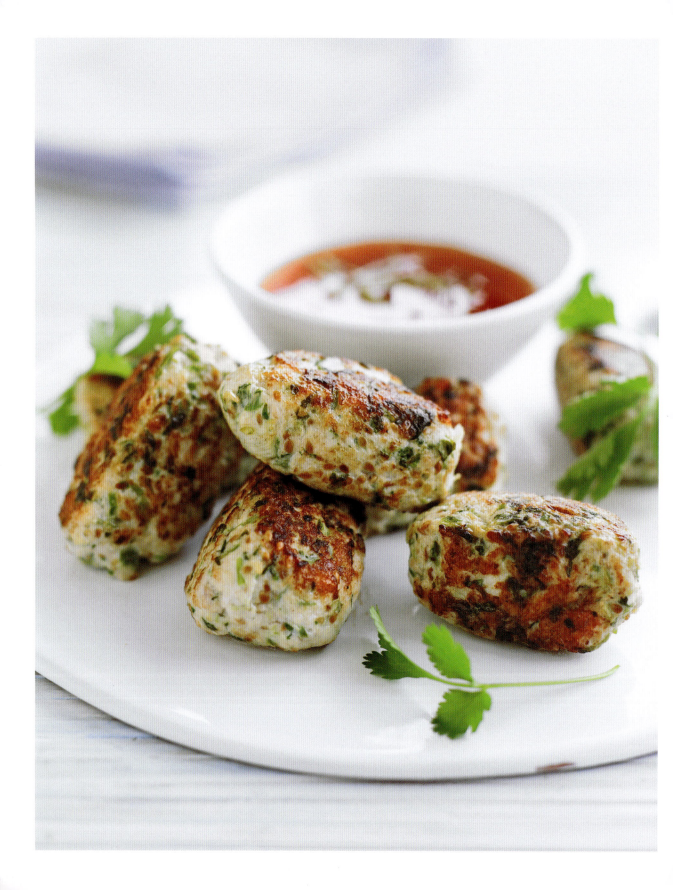

SERVES 4

PREPARATION TIME 15 MINUTES, PLUS CHILLING

COOKING TIME 10 MINUTES

> Sesame seeds are rich in fat-soluble vitamin E, which has antioxidant and anti-inflammatory properties.

sweet chilli chicken patties

- 3 tablespoons sesame seeds
- 4 spring onions
- 15 g (½ oz) fresh coriander, plus extra to garnish
- 500 g (1 lb) minced chicken
- 1 tablespoon light soy sauce
- 3.5 cm (1½ inch) piece of fresh root ginger, peeled and finely grated
- 1 egg white
- 1 tablespoon sesame oil
- 1 tablespoon sunflower oil
- spring onion curls, to garnish (optional)
- 8 tablespoons Thai sweet chilli dipping sauce, to serve

Heat a nonstick frying pan over a medium-low heat and dry-fry the sesame seeds for 2 minutes, stirring frequently, until golden brown and toasted. Set aside.

Place the spring onions and coriander in a food processor and whizz until finely chopped. Alternatively, chop with a knife. Transfer to a bowl and mix with the chicken, toasted sesame seeds, soy sauce, ginger and egg white.

Divide the mixture into 20 mounds on a chopping board, then, using wet hands, shape into slightly flattened rounds. Chill for 1 hour (or longer if you have time).

Heat the sesame and sunflower oils in a large frying pan, add the patties and fry for 10 minutes, turning once or twice, until golden and cooked through to the centre. Arrange on a serving plate and garnish with extra coriander leaves and spring onion curls, if liked. Serve with the chilli dipping sauce.

FOR BABY LEAF STIR-FRY WITH CHILLI, TO SERVE AS AN ACCOMPANIMENT

Heat 2 teaspoons sesame oil in the frying pan, add a 250 g (8 oz) pack ready-prepared baby leaf and baby vegetable stir-fry ingredients and stir-fry for 2–3 minutes until the vegetables are hot. Mix in 2 tablespoons light soy sauce or tamari and 1 tablespoon Thai sweet chilli dipping sauce.

SERVES 4
PREPARATION TIME 10 MINUTES
COOKING TIME 40–45 MINUTES

Butternut soup is low-carb comfort food — perfect if you are managing your blood sugar levels.

butternut & cumin soup

2 tablespoons pumpkin seeds

1 kg (2 lb) butternut squash, peeled, deseeded and chopped

1½ tablespoons olive oil

1 teaspoon dried chilli flakes

2 teaspoons cumin seeds

1 onion, chopped

1 garlic clove, chopped

600 ml (1 pint) hot vegetable stock

2 tablespoons natural yogurt

Heat a nonstick frying pan over a medium-low heat and dry-fry the pumpkin seeds for 2–3 minutes, stirring frequently, until slightly golden and toasted. Set aside.

Place the squash in a roasting tin, drizzle with 1 tablespoon of the oil and sprinkle with the chilli flakes and cumin seeds. Roast in a preheated oven, 200°C (400°F), Gas Mark 6, for 30–35 minutes until tender, tossing occasionally.

Heat the remaining oil in a saucepan, add the onion and garlic and fry for 3–4 minutes. Add the squash and stock and simmer for 5 minutes. Using a hand-held blender, blend the soup until smooth, adding more liquid to loosen, if necessary.

Ladle the soup into 4 bowls and serve topped with dollops of the yogurt and the toasted pumpkin seeds.

FOR ROASTED BUTTERNUT & CUMIN SALAD

Place the butternut squash, cut into wedges, in a roasting tin and add the oil and cumin seeds, omitting the chilli flakes. Roast as above. Toss the roasted squash with 75 g (3 oz) watercress, 12 halved cherry tomatoes, 50 g (2 oz) sugar snap peas and 1 cored, deseeded and sliced red pepper in a serving bowl. Drizzle with 2 tablespoons low-fat dressing and serve.

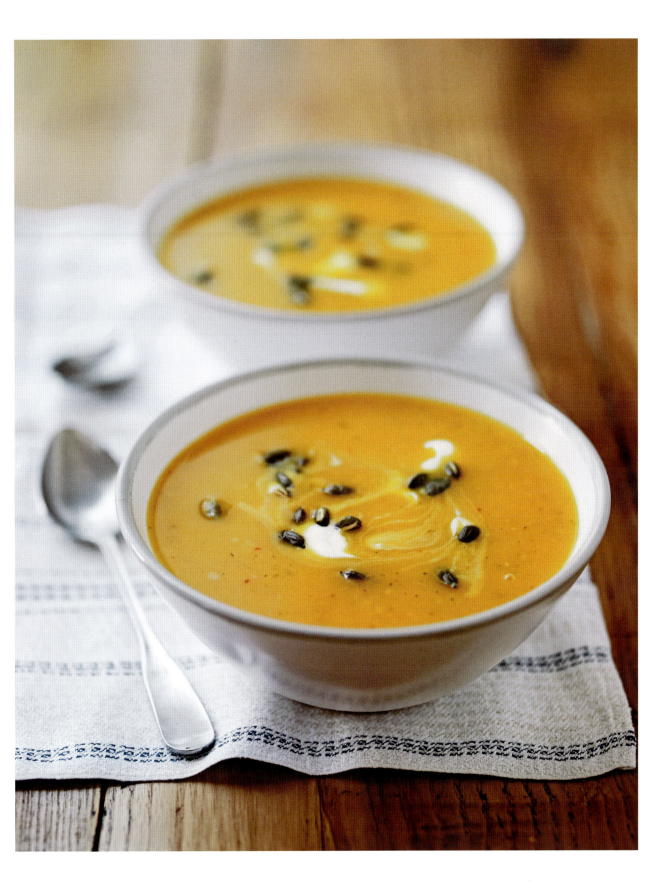

SERVES 4

PREPARATION TIME 20 MINUTES, PLUS COOLING

COOKING TIME 25 MINUTES

mushroom risotto cakes

3 tablespoons olive oil

1 red onion, finely chopped

1 leek, trimmed, cleaned and very finely sliced

250 g (8 oz) chestnut mushrooms, trimmed and roughly chopped

1 garlic clove, crushed

200 g (7 oz) Arborio rice

600 ml (1 pint) vegetable stock, plus extra if needed

150 ml (¼ pint) white wine

75 g (3 oz) polenta

4 tablespoons sunflower oil

dressed salad, to serve

Heat the olive oil in a large, heavy-based frying pan, add the onion, leek, mushrooms and garlic and cook over a medium-high heat for 5–6 minutes until softened and golden in places. Add the rice and stir well, then add the stock and wine, reduce the heat to a gentle simmer and cook, stirring frequently, until the liquid is almost all absorbed and the rice is tender and cooked through, adding more stock if necessary.

Remove the pan from the heat and leave to cool for 20 minutes. The mixture will not only cool but more liquid will be absorbed and the rice will become a little more stodgy.

Divide the mixture into 8 and mould each portion into a large patty, then toss liberally in the polenta and set aside.

Heat the sunflower oil in a frying pan and cook the cakes over a medium-high heat for 2–3 minutes on each side until golden and crisp. Serve hot with a simple dressed salad.

FOR BUTTERNUT SQUASH RISOTTO CAKES

Cook the onion and leek over a medium-high heat as above with 200 g (7 oz) peeled, deseeded and finely chopped butternut squash pieces in place of the mushrooms. Then reduce the heat, cover and cook for a further 3–4 minutes. Remove the lid, add the rice and continue as above. Serve the cakes with a simple salad.

SERVES 4

PREPARATION TIME 10 MINUTES

COOKING TIME 25 MINUTES

Thai-style chicken soup

1 litre (1¾ pints) chicken stock

4 tablespoons Thai fish sauce

1 tablespoon palm sugar or soft light brown sugar

2 lemon grass stalks, sliced in half lengthways

50 g (2 oz) galangal or fresh root ginger, peeled and finely sliced

1 large bunch of fresh coriander, finely chopped, leaves and stalks separated

250 g (8 oz) boneless, skinless chicken thighs, cut into strips

225 g (7½ oz) can bamboo shoots, drained (optional)

200 g (7 oz) vermicelli rice noodles

Put the stock, fish sauce, sugar, lemon grass and galangal or ginger in a large saucepan and bring to the boil, then reduce the heat and simmer gently for 15 minutes. Strain through a sieve to remove the galangal or ginger and lemon grass. Return the liquid to the pan and stir in the chopped coriander stalks.

Add the chicken and simmer gently for a further 4–5 minutes or until cooked through. Add the bamboo shoots, if using.

Meanwhile, put the noodles in a large saucepan of boiling water, turn off the heat and leave to stand for 4 minutes, or according to the packet instructions, until tender. Drain well and divide between deep bowls. Ladle over the chicken soup, sprinkle with the chopped coriander leaves and serve immediately.

SERVES 4

PREPARATION TIME 10 MINUTES

Pumpernickel bread (made with rye) has a low glycaemic index (GI), causing a slower, more gradual rise in blood sugar, which creates less inflammation.

spiced tuna open sandwiches

2 × 250 g (8 oz) cans tuna, drained

4 tablespoons mayonnaise

2 tablespoons sliced celery

¼ teaspoon smoked paprika

¼ teaspoon cayenne pepper

1 tablespoon finely chopped red onion

juice of ½ lemon

¼ cucumber, thinly sliced

4 slices of pumpernickel bread

a few sprigs of watercress

lemon wedges, to serve

Flake the tuna into a bowl, then mix together with the mayonnaise, celery, paprika, cayenne pepper, onion and lemon juice.

Arrange the slices of cucumber on the pumpernickel bread, then top with the tuna mixture. Finish with a few sprigs of watercress.

Serve with lemon wedges.

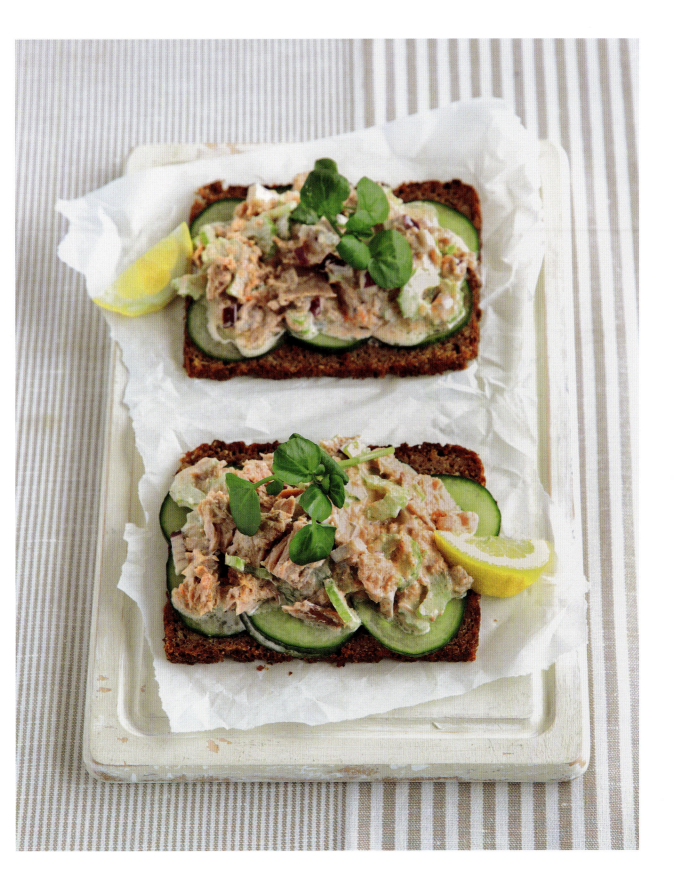

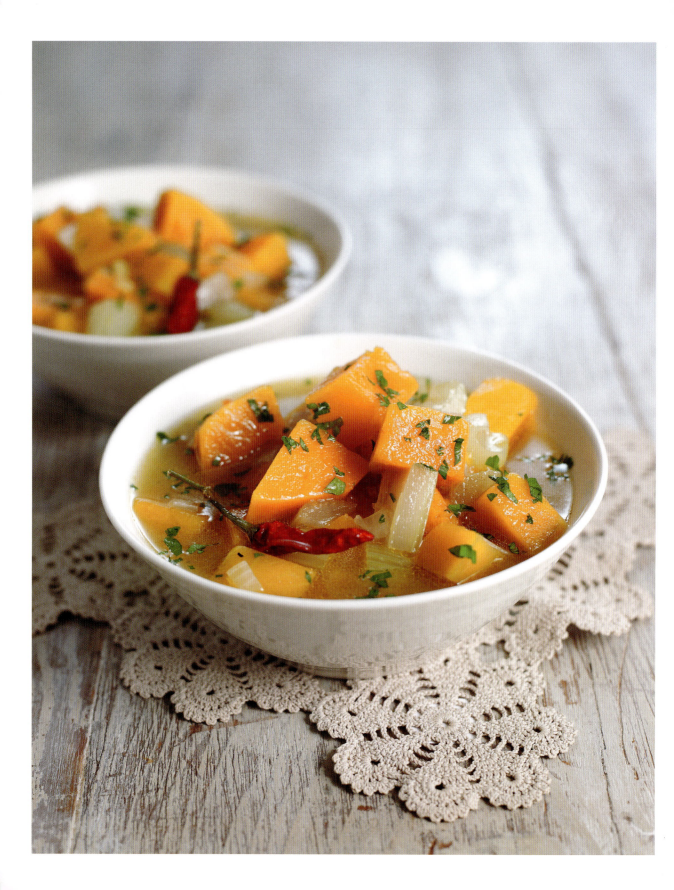

SERVES 4
PREPARATION TIME 15 MINUTES
COOKING TIME 25–30 MINUTES

honeyed pumpkin & ginger broth

2 tablespoons olive oil

15 g (½ oz) butter

1 onion, finely chopped

50 g (2 oz) fresh root ginger, peeled and finely chopped

2 dried red chillies

2–3 celery sticks, cut into bite-sized pieces

700 g (1½ lb) peeled and deseeded pumpkin, cut into bite-sized chunks

1 litre (1¾ pints) hot chicken or vegetable stock

1 small bunch of flat leaf parsley, finely chopped

1–2 tablespoons honey

salt and pepper

Heat the oil and butter in a large, heavy-based saucepan, stir in the onion and ginger and cook for 2–3 minutes until they begin to colour. Add the chillies, celery and pumpkin and cook for 1–2 minutes, stirring to coat well.

Pour in the stock and bring to the boil, then reduce the heat and cook gently for 20–25 minutes until the vegetables are tender. Season and stir in most of the parsley.

Meanwhile, in a small saucepan, gently heat the honey until it begins to bubble. Ladle the broth into serving bowls, drizzle over the hot honey and garnish with the remaining parsley.

SERVES 4
PREPARATION TIME 5 MINUTES
COOKING TIME 10 MINUTES

ciabatta toasties with Mediterranean vegetables

5 tablespoons olive oil, plus extra for drizzling

½ aubergine, trimmed and thinly sliced

1 ciabatta loaf

4 tablespoons pesto (see page 32)

1 large beef tomato, thinly sliced

4 slices of mozzarella cheese

pepper

Heat the oil in a large, heavy-based frying pan and cook the aubergine slices in batches over a high heat for 1–2 minutes on each side until browned and tender. Remove with a fish slice and keep warm.

Meanwhile, cut the ciabatta loaf in half lengthways, then each half in half again widthways. Place on the grill rack and cook under a preheated hot grill, cut-side up, for 1 minute until golden.

Spread each ciabatta toastie with 1 tablespoon of the pesto. Top with the warm aubergine slices, then the tomato slices and finally the mozzarella slices. Drizzle each toastie with 1 tablespoon olive oil, then return to the grill and cook for a further 2 minutes until the mozzarella is melting and beginning to brown in places.

Season with pepper and serve warm.

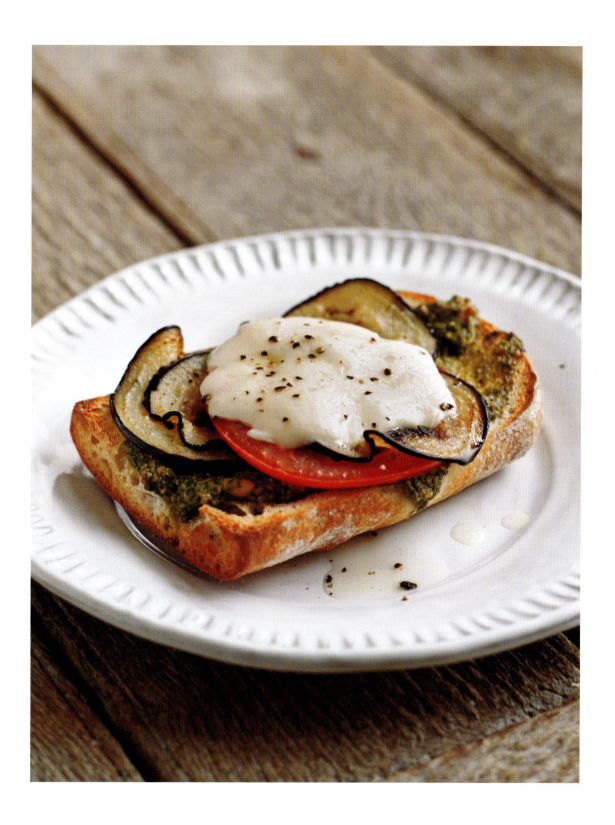

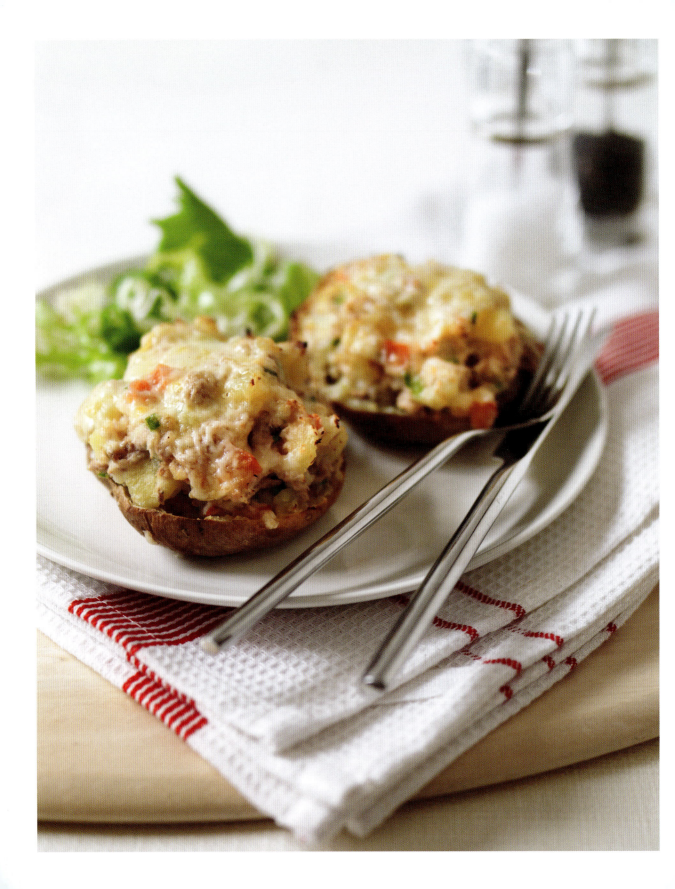

SERVES 4

PREPARATION TIME 10 MINUTES, PLUS COOLING

COOKING TIME 1 HOUR 5 MINUTES

> Eating the skin of a baked potato provides extra fibre and vitamin C, and helps maintain stable blood sugar levels compared to eating only the flesh.

tuna & jalapeño baked potatoes

4 large baking potatoes

2 × 160 g (5½ oz) cans tuna in spring water, drained

2 tablespoons drained and chopped green jalapeño peppers in brine

2 spring onions, finely chopped

4 firm, ripe tomatoes, deseeded and chopped

2 tablespoons chopped chives

3 tablespoons soured cream

100 g (3½ oz) reduced-fat extra mature Cheddar cheese, grated

salt and pepper

frisée salad, to serve

Prick the potatoes all over with the tip of a sharp knife and place directly in a preheated oven, 180°C (350°F), Gas Mark 4, for 1 hour or until crisp on the outside and the insides are tender. Leave until cool enough to handle.

Cut the potatoes in half and scoop the cooked flesh into a bowl. Place the empty potato skins, cut side up, on a baking sheet. Mix the tuna, jalapeño peppers, spring onions, tomatoes and chives into the potato in the bowl. Gently fold in the soured cream, then season with salt and pepper to taste.

Spoon the filling into the potato skins, sprinkle with the Cheddar and cook under a preheated medium-hot grill for 4–5 minutes or until hot and melted. Serve immediately with a frisée salad.

FOR SPICY TUNA WRAPS

Spoon 4 tablespoons chunky spicy tomato salsa on to 4 large, wholemeal flour tortillas. Scatter with the tuna, jalapeño peppers and spring onions. Omit the tomatoes, chives and Cheddar and top with ½ shredded iceberg lettuce. Roll up the wraps tightly and cut in half diagonally. Serve with a little low-fat soured cream, if liked.

SERVES 4

PREPARATION TIME 25 MINUTES

If you keep a batch of these veggies in the refrigerator, their gut-loving probiotic benefits will develop over time.

mixed pickled vegetables

1 small cucumber

1 teaspoon salt

2 carrots, peeled

1 large white radish, peeled

1 red pepper, cored and deseeded

2 tablespoons blanched almonds

2 teaspoons pink peppercorns

1–2 teaspoons cumin seeds

pinch of saffron threads

1–2 cinnamon sticks

juice of 2 lemons

1–2 tablespoons cider vinegar

1 tablespoon granulated sugar

1–2 tablespoons orange blossom water

2 tablespoons finely chopped fresh coriander

Peel and deseed the cucumber, then cut into matchsticks and place in a colander, sprinkle with the salt and leave to stand for 5 minutes. Rinse, drain and pat dry, then place in a large, non-metallic bowl.

Cut the carrots, radish and red pepper into matchsticks. Add to the cucumber with the almonds and spices, then stir in the lemon juice, vinegar, sugar and orange blossom water. Cover and chill for 15–20 minutes. Just before serving, toss in the coriander.

The pickles can also be stored in a sterilized jar, sealed with a vinegar-proof lid, in the refrigerator for 3–4 weeks.

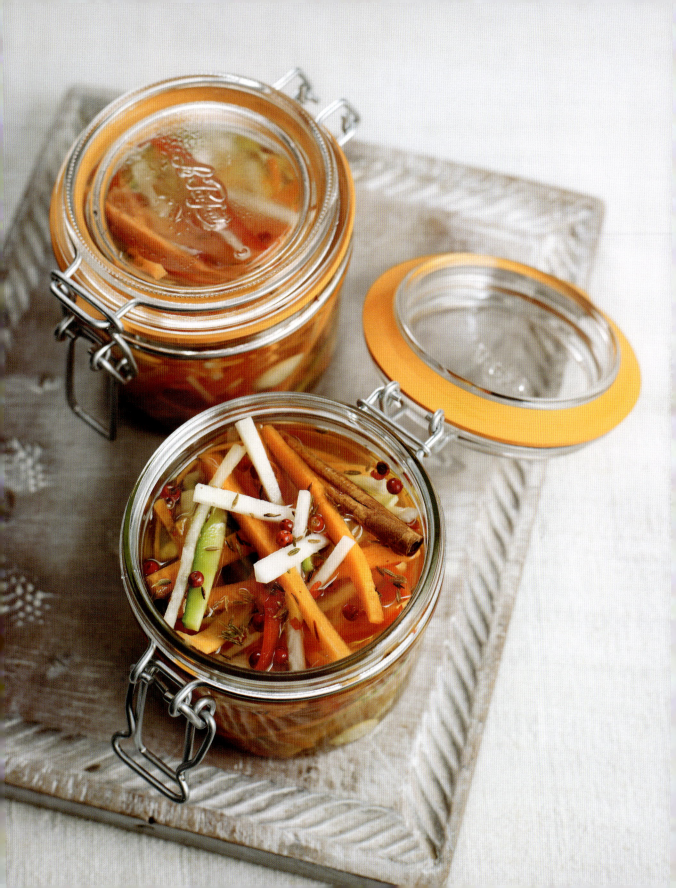

SERVES 4
PREPARATION TIME 10 MINUTES
COOKING TIME 15–20 MINUTES

> Garlic contains sulphur compounds that have been found to benefit the immune system and inhibit triggers of the inflammatory response, including cytokines.

sweet potato & garlic mash

- 1 kg (2 lb) sweet potatoes, peeled and cut into 2.5 cm (1 inch) pieces
- 4–6 smoked garlic cloves, peeled but left whole
- 25 g (1 oz) salted butter
- 2 tablespoons milk
- 2 tablespoons chopped flat leaf parsley
- salt and pepper

Place the sweet potatoes and smoked garlic cloves in a large saucepan, cover with cold water and bring to the boil. Reduce the heat and simmer for 10–12 minutes until tender, then drain well.

Return the sweet potatoes and garlic to the pan and mash until smooth.

Set the pan over a low heat, then push the mash to one side, add the butter to the base of the pan and leave to melt. Pour the milk on to the butter and heat for 1–2 minutes, then beat into the mash.

Stir in the parsley, season to taste with salt and pepper and serve.

FOR SWEET POTATO, CHEESE & MUSTARD MASH

Cook the potatoes as above, omitting the smoked garlic, then beat in the butter and milk with 2 tablespoons wholegrain mustard and 125 g (4 oz) grated mature Cheddar cheese. Stir in 2 tablespoons chopped chives, season to taste with salt and pepper and serve.

SERVES 4
PREPARATION TIME 5 MINUTES
COOKING TIME ABOUT 35 MINUTES

Lentils provide protein, fibre and phytochemicals. Using them in place of animal proteins significantly lowers your body's overall inflammation burden.

spiced green lentils with tomatoes

- 2 tablespoons argan oil
- 2 onions, finely chopped
- 4 garlic cloves, finely chopped
- 2 teaspoons ground turmeric
- 2 teaspoons ground fenugreek
- 225 g (7½ oz) dried green lentils, rinsed, picked over and drained
- 400 g (13 oz) can chopped tomatoes
- 2 teaspoons sugar
- 750 ml (1¼ pints) water
- 1 small bunch of fresh coriander, finely chopped
- salt and pepper

Heat the oil in the base of a tagine or a large, heavy-based saucepan over a medium heat, stir in the onions and garlic and cook for 2–3 minutes to soften a little. Add the turmeric, fenugreek and lentils and stir to coat well, then stir in the tomatoes and sugar.

Pour in the measured water and bring to the boil, then reduce the heat, cover and cook gently for about 30 minutes until the lentils are tender but not mushy, adding a little more water if necessary. Stir in half the coriander and season with salt and pepper. Scatter over the remaining coriander and serve as side dish to grilled or roasted meat and poultry.

FOR YELLOW SPIT PEAS WITH TOMATOES & GINGER

Replace the lentils with 225 g (7½ oz) yellow split peas. Follow the recipe above, adding 40 g (1½ oz) fresh root ginger, peeled and finely chopped, to the tagine or saucepan with the onions and garlic, cook for 2–3 minutes, then stir in the turmeric and split peas and proceed as above.

LIGHT BITES & SIDES

SERVES 4

PREPARATION TIME 2 MINUTES

COOKING TIME 8 MINUTES

baby vegetables with pesto

200 g (7 oz) baby courgettes, halved lengthways

125 g (4 oz) baby leeks, halved lengthways

150 g (5 oz) baby carrots, halved lengthways

100 g (3½ oz) trimmed asparagus spears

2 tablespoons olive oil

2 tablespoons lemon juice

4 tablespoons pesto (see page 32)

salt and pepper

focaccia (see page 101), to serve

Place all the vegetables in a large bowl and add the oil. Season to taste and stir gently to coat.

Heat a large griddle pan over a high heat, add half the vegetables and cook for about 2 minutes on each side until lightly charred. Remove from the pan and keep warm while you cook the remaining vegetables in the same way.

Divide the vegetables between 4 serving plates, drizzle with the lemon juice, then spoon the pesto over them. Serve immediately with focaccia.

FOR PEA & PESTO SOUP

Place 750 ml (1¼ pints) boiling vegetable stock in a large saucepan. Add 450 g (14½ oz) frozen peas and simmer for 5 minutes until tender. Use a hand-held blender or food processor to blend the soup until smooth. Return to the pan, stir in 2 tablespoons crème fraîche and 2 tablespoons fresh pesto (see page 32). Heat through, season to taste and serve immediately with crusty bread.

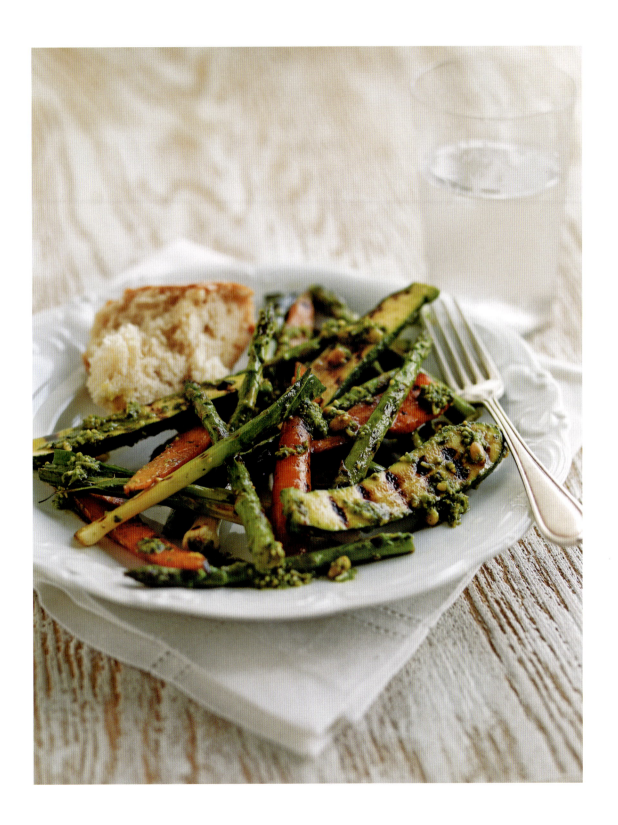

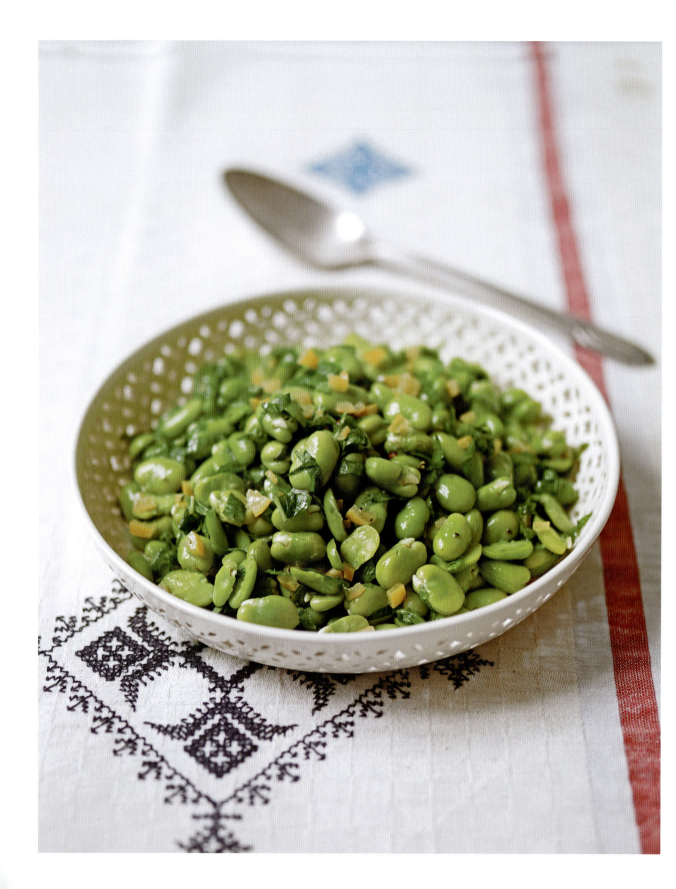

SERVES 4
PREPARATION TIME 15 MINUTES
COOKING TIME 4–5 MINUTES

> Fresh herbs like mint contain lots of vitamin C and beneficial plant-based antioxidants that are powerful components of an anti-inflammatory diet.

broad beans with mint & lemon

750 g (1½ lb) fresh or frozen broad beans, podded

2 tablespoons olive oil

juice of 1 lemon

finely chopped rind of 1 preserved lemon

1 bunch of mint, finely shredded

salt and pepper

Fill a large saucepan with water and bring it to the boil. Add the broad beans, return to the boil and cook for 3–4 minutes until tender. Drain the beans, refresh under cold running water and transfer to a bowl.

Add the olive oil, lemon juice, most of the preserved lemon rind and mint to the bowl with the broad beans. Toss well and season with salt and pepper. Garnish with the remaining preserved lemon rind and mint. Serve as a side salad to accompany tagines.

SERVES 4
PREPARATION TIME 5 MINUTES
COOKING TIME 25 MINUTES

roasted spiced pumpkin

2 teaspoons coriander seeds

2 teaspoons cumin seeds

2–3 garlic cloves

1–2 teaspoons sea salt

1 teaspoon finely chopped dried red chilli or cayenne pepper

1 teaspoon ground cinnamon

1 teaspoon ground allspice

3 tablespoons olive or argan oil

1 small pumpkin, halved, deseeded and cut into thin wedges

Using a pestle and mortar, pound the coriander and cumin seeds, garlic and salt to form a coarse paste. Stir in the chilli or cayenne, cinnamon and allspice, then mix in the oil.

Rub the mixture over the pumpkin wedges, then place, skin side down, in a roasting tin or ovenproof dish. Roast in a preheated oven, 200°C (400°F), Gas Mark 6, for 25 minutes until tender. Serve with grilled or roasted meat dishes.

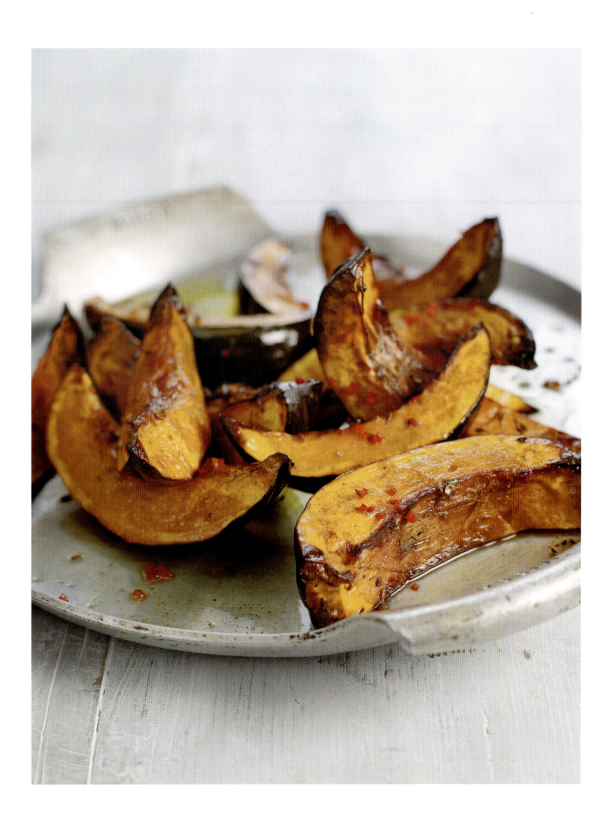

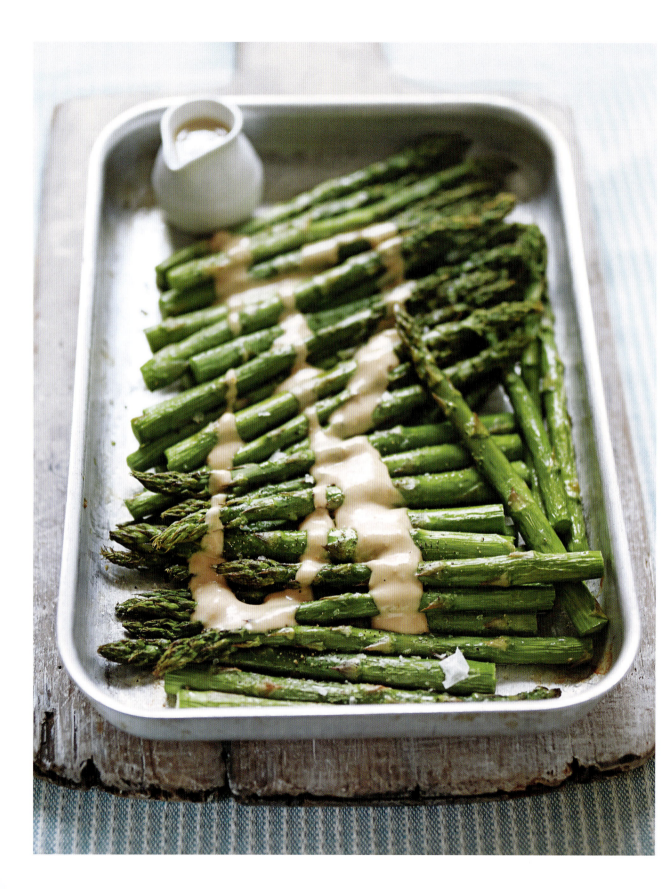

SERVES 4

PREPARATION TIME 15 MINUTES

COOKING TIME 15 MINUTES

The folate in asparagus helps reduce levels of homocysteine, an amino acid linked to inflammation and cardiovascular diseases.

asparagus with sesame dressing

3 bunches of asparagus spears, trimmed

4 tablespoons olive oil

FOR THE DRESSING

4 tablespoons sesame seeds

4 tablespoons tahini

finely grated rind and juice of 1 lemon

3 tablespoons light soy sauce

2 tablespoons mirin

4 tablespoons water

Lay the asparagus spears in a roasting tin, drizzle with 2 tablespoons of the oil and toss until evenly coated in the oil. Roast in a preheated oven, 220°C (425°F), Gas Mark 7, for 15 minutes until tender and lightly charred in places.

Meanwhile, toast the sesame seeds in a dry frying pan over a medium heat, shaking the pan occasionally, for about 2 minutes until golden. Transfer to a jug with the tahini, lemon rind and juice, soy sauce, mirin and the measured water. Add the remaining olive oil, then use a stick blender to blend until smooth.

Spoon half the dressing over the roasted asparagus and toss well to coat. Arrange on 4 serving plates and serve the remaining dressing on the side.

SERVES 4
PREPARATION TIME 20 MINUTES
COOKING TIME 30–35 MINUTES

> Whole olives provide a polyphenol called oleocanthal which inhibits the activity of enzymes that promote inflammation (similar to how ibuprofen works).

sweet potatoes with green olives

3–4 tablespoons olive or argan oil

1 onion, coarsely chopped

25 g (1 oz) fresh root ginger, peeled and grated

1–2 teaspoons cumin seeds

500 g (1 lb) sweet potatoes, peeled and cut into bite-sized pieces

juice of 1 lemon

12 large cracked green olives

2–3 tablespoons orange blossom water

1 small bunch of fresh coriander, finely chopped

salt and pepper

Heat the oil in the base of a tagine or a large, heavy-based saucepan over a medium heat, stir in the onion, ginger and cumin seeds and cook for 2–3 minutes until the onion starts to soften. Add the sweet potatoes and stir to coat well.

Pour in the lemon juice, then cover and cook gently for 15 minutes. Add the olives and the orange blossom water, re-cover and cook for a further 10–15 minutes to let the flavours mingle. Season to taste with salt and pepper, then stir in the coriander. Serve with couscous, if liked, or as an accompaniment to a meat or poultry tagine.

FOR GREEN OLIVES WITH TOMATOES & PRESERVED LEMON

Heat 2 tablespoons olive oil in the base of a tagine or heavy-based saucepan over a medium heat, stir in 1 finely chopped onion, 2 finely chopped garlic cloves and 2 teaspoons coriander seeds and cook for 2–3 minutes to let the flavours mingle. Toss in 16 large cracked green olives and add 1 × 400 g (13 oz) can chopped tomatoes and 1–2 teaspoons sugar. Cover and cook gently for 15 minutes. Season to taste with salt and pepper, then stir in 1 small bunch of finely chopped coriander. Serve as an accompaniment to meat and poultry tagines.

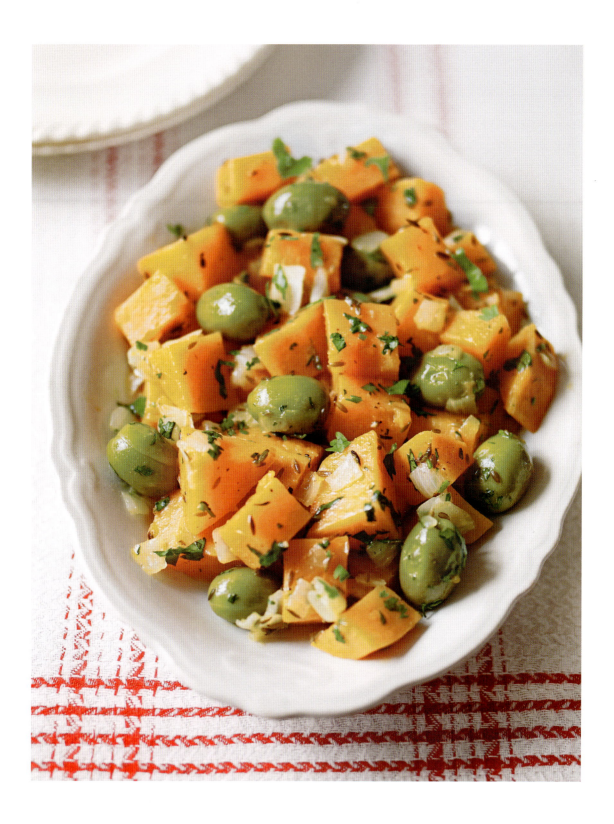

Something Sweet

194	**tropical fruit cake**
197	**rice pudding**
198	**fig & honey pots**
199	**vanilla-spiced fruit salad**
201	**autumn fruit oaty crumble**
202	**chewy nutty chocolate brownies**
205	**creamy mango & passion fruit**
206	**mixed berry salad**
209	**rich chocolate mousse**
210	**summer berry sorbet**
213	**strawberry & lavender crush**
214	**stem ginger & dark choc cookies**
217	**perfect pecan pies**
218	**chocolate & chestnut roulade**

SERVES 12

PREPARATION TIME 15 MINUTES, PLUS COOLING

COOKING TIME 1 HOUR–1 HOUR 10 MINUTES

Dried fruit is a good source of anaemic-protective iron and fibre for a healthy gut.

tropical fruit cake

100 g (3½ oz) raisins

250 g (8 oz) mixed soft dried tropical fruit, such as pineapple, mango, papaya and apricots, cut into small pieces

1 teaspoon mixed spice

1 teaspoon ground ginger

125 g (4 oz) unsalted butter, cubed

125 g (4 oz) soft light brown sugar

150 ml (¼ pint) cold water

225 g (7½ oz) self-raising flour

1 egg, lightly beaten

Grease and line the base of a 1 kg (2 lb) loaf tin with nonstick baking paper (or use a loaf tin liner).

Place the raisins, dried tropical fruit, mixed spice, ginger, butter, sugar and measured water in a saucepan. Warm over a low heat until the butter has melted, stirring occasionally with a wooden spoon, then bring to the boil.

Boil the fruit mixture for 5 minutes, then remove from the heat and leave to cool in the pan.

Stir the flour and beaten egg into the cooled fruit mixture until well combined, then spoon into the prepared tin.

Bake in the centre of a preheated oven, 150°C (300°F), Gas Mark 2, for 50 minutes–1 hour or until a skewer inserted into the centre comes out clean.

Leave the cake to cool in the tin, then cut into slices to serve.

FOR TRADITIONAL FRUIT CAKE

Follow the recipe above to make the cake mixture, using a mixture of currants, chopped soft dried pitted dates, sultanas and glacé cherries in place of the dried tropical fruit and omitting the ground ginger. Bake as above.

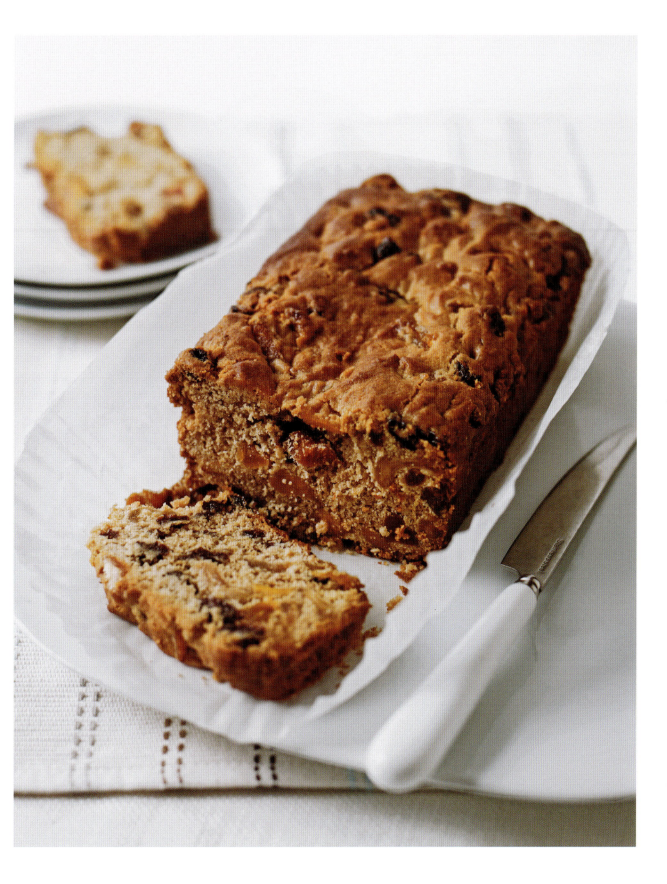

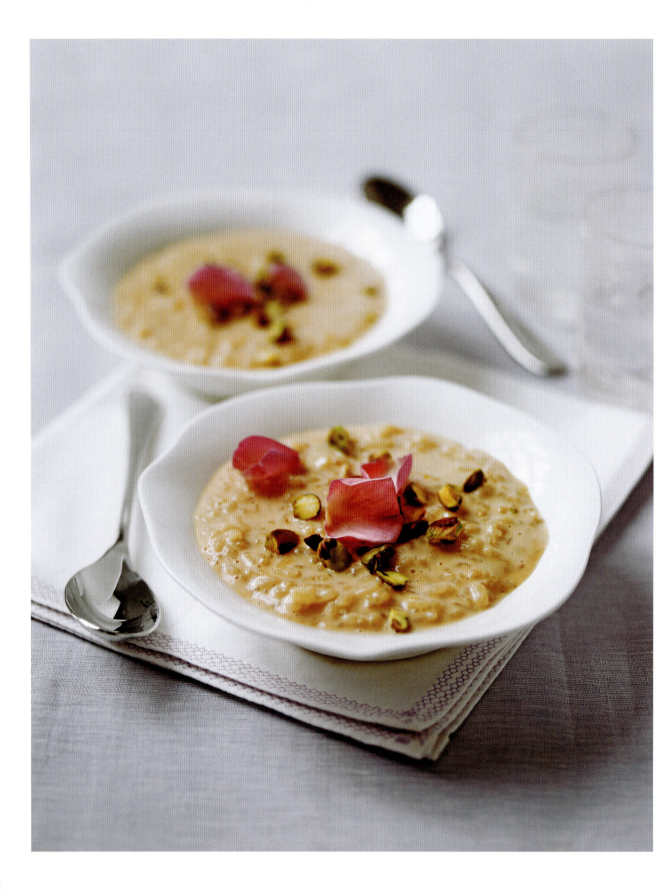

SERVES 4
PREPARATION TIME 5 MINUTES
COOKING TIME 30 MINUTES

rice pudding

100 g (3½ oz) pudding rice, rinsed and drained

50 g (2 oz) caster sugar

2 cinnamon sticks

1 teaspoon vanilla bean paste

450 ml (¾ pint) water

400 g (13 oz) can evaporated milk

2 teaspoons rosewater

50 g (2 oz) pistachio nuts, roughly chopped

a few edible rose petals (optional)

Place the rice, sugar, cinnamon sticks, vanilla bean paste and measured water in a saucepan and bring to the boil.

Reduce the heat and simmer the rice, uncovered, for 20 minutes. Stir in the evaporated milk and rosewater and simmer for a further 10 minutes until the rice is tender. Remove the cinnamon sticks.

Pour the rice pudding into warmed serving dishes and sprinkle with the pistachios and rose petals, if liked. Serve immediately.

FOR ORANGE & CARDAMOM RICE PUDDING

Place the rinsed and drained pudding rice, the caster sugar, measured water, the grated rind and juice of 1 orange and 6 crushed cardamom pods in a saucepan. Bring to the boil, then reduce the heat and simmer for 25 minutes. Stir in the evaporated milk and cook for a further 5 minutes until the rice is tender. Serve decorated with toasted flaked almonds.

SERVES 4

PREPARATION TIME 10 MINUTES, PLUS CHILLING

> Fresh figs contain polyphenols which improve the health of anti-inflammatory bacteria in our microbiome.

fig & honey pots

6 ripe fresh figs, thinly sliced, plus 2 extra (optional), cut into wedges, to decorate

450 ml (¾ pint) Greek yogurt

4 tablespoons clear honey

2 tablespoons chopped pistachio nuts

Arrange the fig slices snugly in the bottom of 4 glasses or glass bowls. Spoon the yogurt over the figs and chill in the refrigerator for 10–15 minutes.

Drizzle 1 tablespoon honey over each dessert and sprinkle the pistachio nuts on top. Decorate with the wedges of fig, if liked, before serving.

FOR HOT FIGS WITH HONEY

Heat a griddle pan or large frying pan over a medium-high heat and, when hot, add 8 whole ripe fresh figs and cook for 8 minutes, turning occasionally, until charred on the outside. Alternatively, cook under a preheated hot grill. Remove and cut in half. Divide between serving plates, top each with 1 tablespoon Greek yogurt and drizzle with a little clear honey.

SERVES 4

PREPARATION TIME 10 MINUTES, PLUS COOLING

COOKING TIME 4–5 MINUTES

A spectrum of bright fruit colours is always a good signifier of antioxidant and anti-inflammatory potential.

vanilla-spiced fruit salad

150 ml (¼ pint) apple juice

1 vanilla pod, split in half lengthways

2 kiwi ruit, peeled and sliced

250 g (8 oz) strawberries, hulled and thickly sliced

125 g (4 oz) blueberries

1 mango, peeled, stoned and sliced

mint leaves, to decorate

Warm the apple juice in a small saucepan with the split vanilla pod over a medium-low heat. Simmer gently for 4–5 minutes, then leave to cool completely. Remove the vanilla pod and scrape the seeds into the light syrup.

Combine the fruits in a large bowl and drizzle over the vanilla-spiced juice. Stir gently to coat and spoon into serving bowls. Sprinkle with mint leaves and serve.

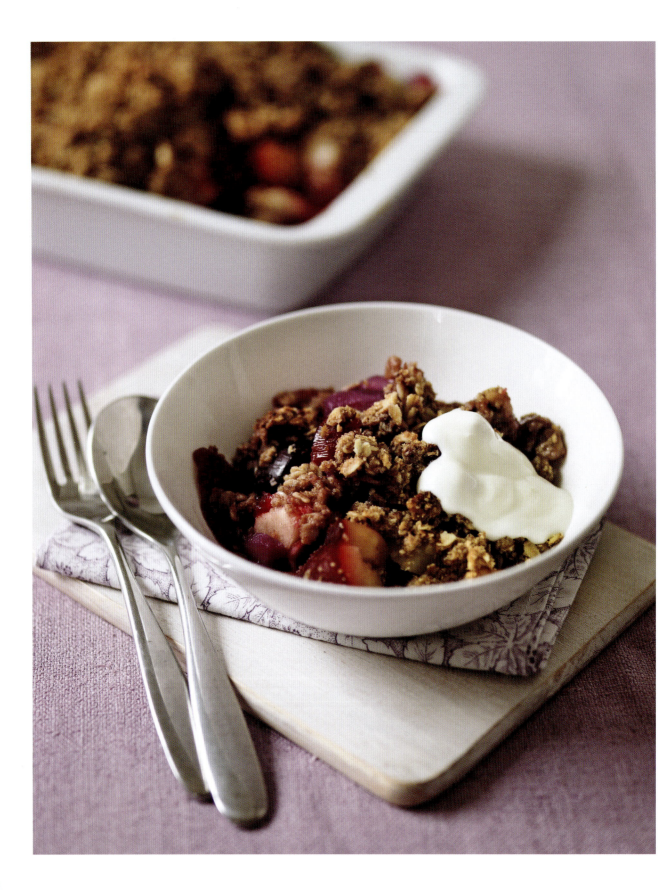

SERVES 4

PREPARATION TIME 15 MINUTES

COOKING TIME 40–45 MINUTES

This oaty fruit crumble counts as more than one of your five-a-day and is a good source of fibre.

autumn fruit oaty crumble

1 dessert apple, peeled, cored and sliced

25 g (1 oz) ready-to-eat dried apples, chopped (optional)

400 g (13 oz) can pear halves in juice, drained with 4 tablespoons juice reserved, roughly chopped

200 g (7 oz) ripe plums, halved, stoned and quartered

25 g (1 oz) raisins or golden raisins

fat-free Greek yogurt, to serve (optional)

TOPPING

75 g (3 oz) wholemeal flour

50 g (2 oz) rolled oats

25 g (1 oz) bran

pinch of salt

50 g (2 oz) pecan nuts, chopped

2 tablespoons soft dark brown sugar

¾ teaspoon mixed spice

75 g (3 oz) butter, melted

Put all of the prepared fruit and raisins into a shallow, rectangular ovenproof dish, approximately 28 x 20 cm (11 x 8 inches). Drizzle over the reserved pear juice.

Mix together the dry topping ingredients in a large bowl. Pour over the melted butter and combine until the mixture resembles large breadcrumbs. Sprinkle over the fruit and press down firmly.

Place in a preheated oven, 180°C (350°F), Gas Mark 4, for 40–45 minutes or until golden and crisp. Serve with fat-free Greek yogurt, if liked.

FOR FOREST FRUIT & CLEMENTINE CRUMBLE

Replace the fresh and dried fruits with 450 g (14 ½ oz) frozen forest fruits, thawed and drained of excess liquid. Slice 2 clementines into segments, discarding the pith, and mix with the forest fruits. Spread the fruit over the base of the ovenproof dish, cover with the crumble topping and bake as above.

MAKES 15
PREPARATION TIME 10 MINUTES
COOKING TIME 30 MINUTES

Flavanols and theobromine in dark chocolate help maintain healthy blood pressure and blood vessel function.

chewy nutty chocolate brownies

75 g (3 oz) plain dark chocolate, broken into pieces

100 g (3½ oz) butter, plus extra for greasing

200 g (7 oz) soft light brown sugar

2 eggs, beaten

few drops of vanilla extract

50 g (2 oz) ground almonds

25 g (1 oz) brown rice flour

150 g (5 oz) mixed nuts, toasted and roughly chopped

vanilla ice cream, to serve

Grease and line a 28 x 18 cm (11 x 7 inch) baking tin.

Place the chocolate and butter in a large heatproof bowl over a saucepan of simmering water (do not let the bowl touch the water) and leave until melted. Stir in all the remaining ingredients and combine well.

Pour the mixture into the prepared tin and place in a preheated oven, 180°C (350°F), Gas Mark 4, for 30 minutes until slightly springy in the centre.

Remove from the oven and leave to cool for 10 minutes in the tin, then cut into 15 squares. Serve with a generous dollop of vanilla ice cream.

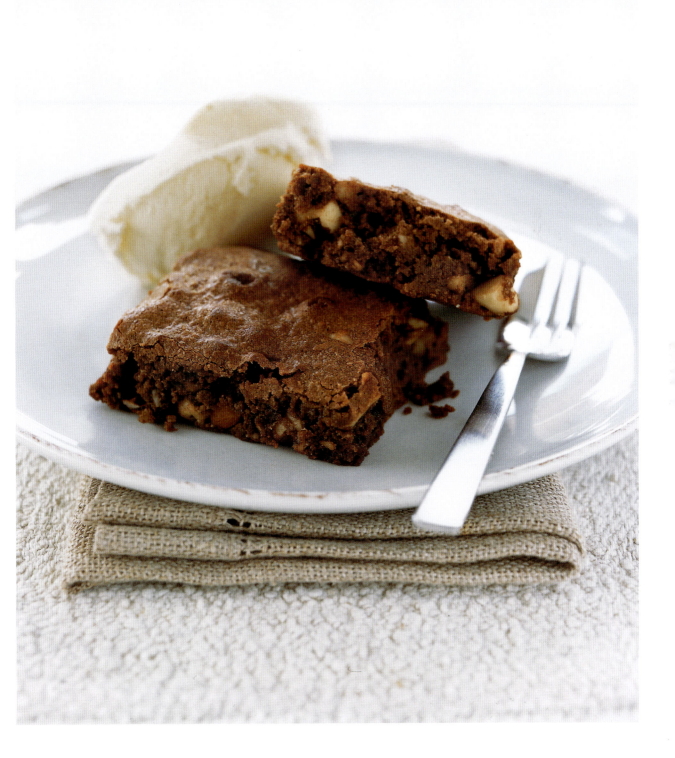

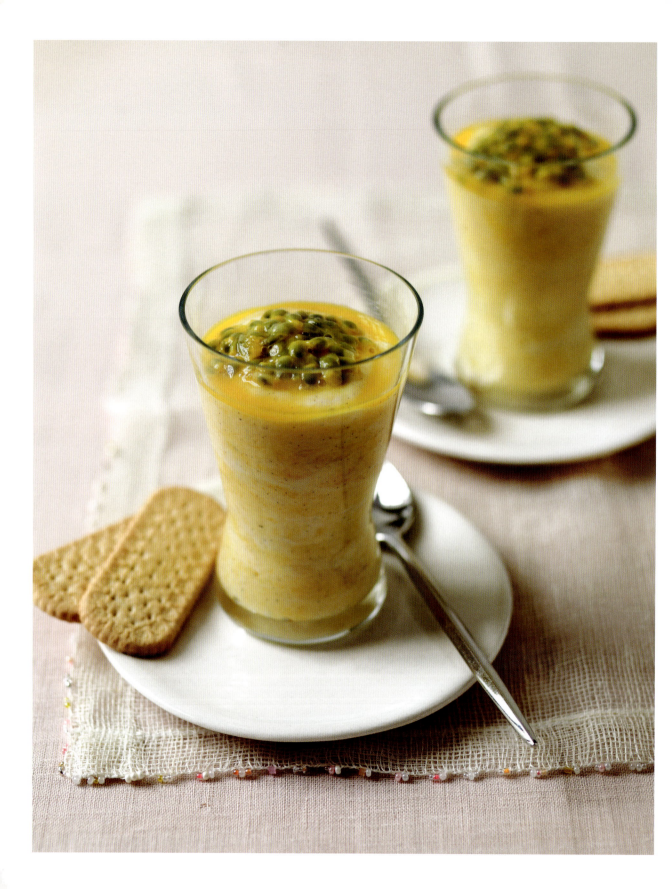

SERVES 4

PREPARATION TIME 10 MINUTES

> Mangoes are rich in the antioxidant vitamins C, A and E, which reduce inflammation by neutralizing free radicals. In addition, this dessert bumps up your intake of bone-friendly calcium.

creamy mango & passion fruit

1 large mango, peeled, stoned and cut into chunks

750 ml (1¼ pints) fat-free natural yogurt

1–2 tablespoons agave nectar, to taste

1 vanilla pod, split in half lengthways

4 passion fruit, halved

thin biscuits, to serve (optional)

Place the mango in a food processor or blender and blend to a purée.

Put the yogurt and agave nectar, according to taste, in a large bowl, scrape in the seeds from the vanilla pod and beat together. Gently fold in the mango purée and spoon into tall glasses or glass serving dishes.

Scoop the seeds from the passion fruit and spoon over the mango yogurt. Serve immediately with thin biscuits, if liked.

FOR BLACKCURRANT & ALMOND YOGURT

Purée 250 g (8 oz) blackcurrants as above and fold into the yogurt with the agave nectar, according to taste, and 1 teaspoon almond essence. Spoon into tall, glass serving dishes and scatter with toasted almonds, to serve.

SERVES 4–6

PREPARATION TIME 10 MINUTES

Packed with fibre and polyphenols, berries promote the health of your intestinal bacteria.

mixed berry salad

400 g (13 oz) strawberries

250 g (8 oz) raspberries

150 g (5 oz) blueberries

150 g (5 oz) blackberries

1 small bunch of mint, finely chopped, plus a few sprigs to decorate

3 tablespoons elderflower syrup

Hull and halve the strawberries. Wash all the berries and drain well.

Put the berries in a large serving bowl and add the chopped mint and elderflower syrup. Mix together carefully and serve, decorated with extra mint sprigs.

FOR WARM BERRY SALAD

Dilute 100 ml (3½ fl oz) elderflower syrup in 600 ml (1 pint) water, add 50 g (2 oz) caster sugar and bring to the boil in a heavy-based saucepan. Add the berries, prepared as above, to the pan and turn off the heat. Let the berries cool slightly, then serve with half-fat crème fraîche. The berries will keep for up to 5 days in the syrup in the refrigerator.

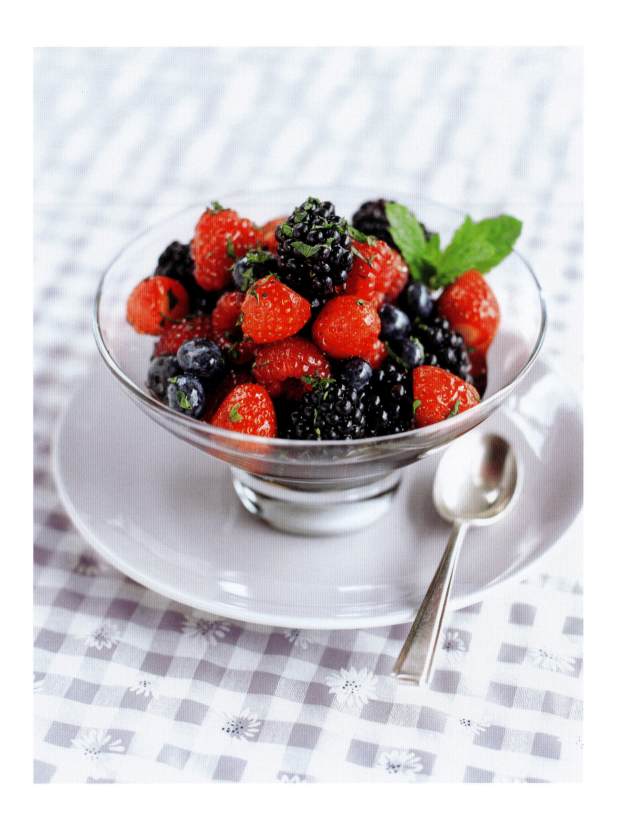

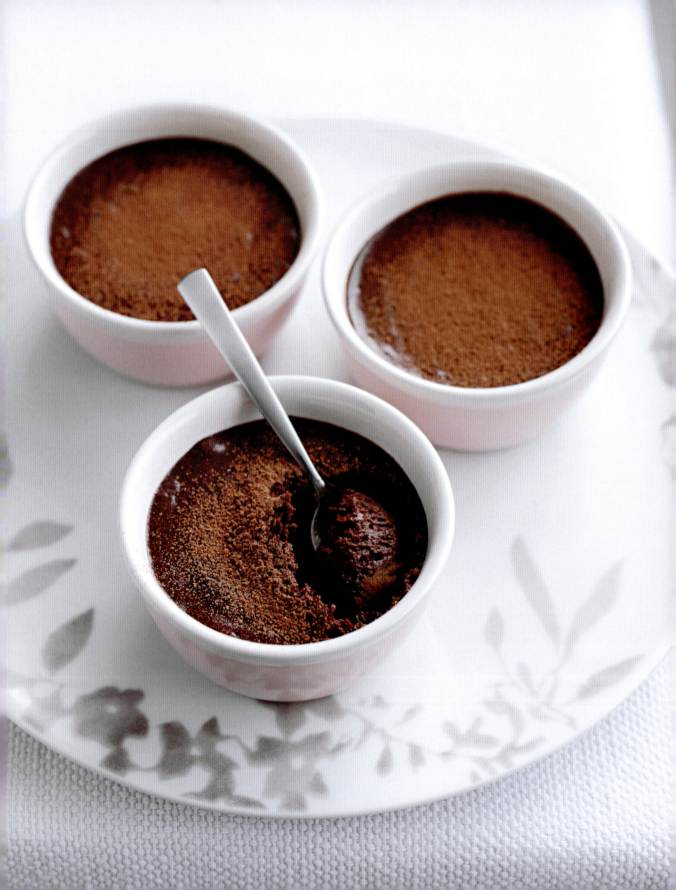

SERVES 4
PREPARATION TIME 5 MINUTES, PLUS CHILLING
COOKING TIME 3–4 MINUTES

> For the biggest antioxidant health benefits (and higher amounts of fibre and minerals) choose chocolate with minimum 70% cocoa.

rich chocolate mousse

175 g (6 oz) plain dark chocolate, broken into pieces

100 ml (3½ fl oz) double cream

3 eggs, separated

cocoa powder, for dusting

Put the chocolate and cream in a heatproof bowl set over a saucepan of gently simmering water (do not let the bowl touch the water) and stir until the chocolate has melted. Leave to cool for 5 minutes, then beat in the egg yolks one at a time.

Whisk the egg whites in a separate clean bowl until stiff, then lightly fold into the chocolate mixture until combined. Spoon the mousse into 4 dessert glasses or cups and chill for 2 hours. Dust with cocoa powder before serving.

FOR CHOCOLATE & ORANGE MOUSSE

Follow the recipe above but add the grated rind of 1 large orange and 2 tablespoons Grand Marnier to the melted chocolate and cream. Continue the recipe as above.

SERVES 2

PREPARATION TIME 5 MINUTES, PLUS FREEZING

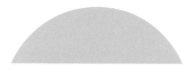

Frozen berries are as nutritious as fresh — and may even have more vitamin C.

summer berry sorbet

250 g (8 oz) frozen mixed summer berries

75 ml (3 fl oz) spiced berry cordial

2 tablespoons Kirsch

1 tablespoon lime juice

Put a shallow plastic container in the freezer to chill. Process the frozen berries, cordial, Kirsch and lime juice in a food processor or blender to a smooth purée. Be careful not to over-process, as this will soften the mixture too much.

Spoon into the chilled container and freeze for at least 25 minutes. Spoon into serving bowls and serve.

FOR RASPBERRY SORBET

Replace the main recipe ingredients with frozen raspberries, elderflower cordial, crème de cassis and lemon juice. Use the same quantities and method as the summer berry sorbet.

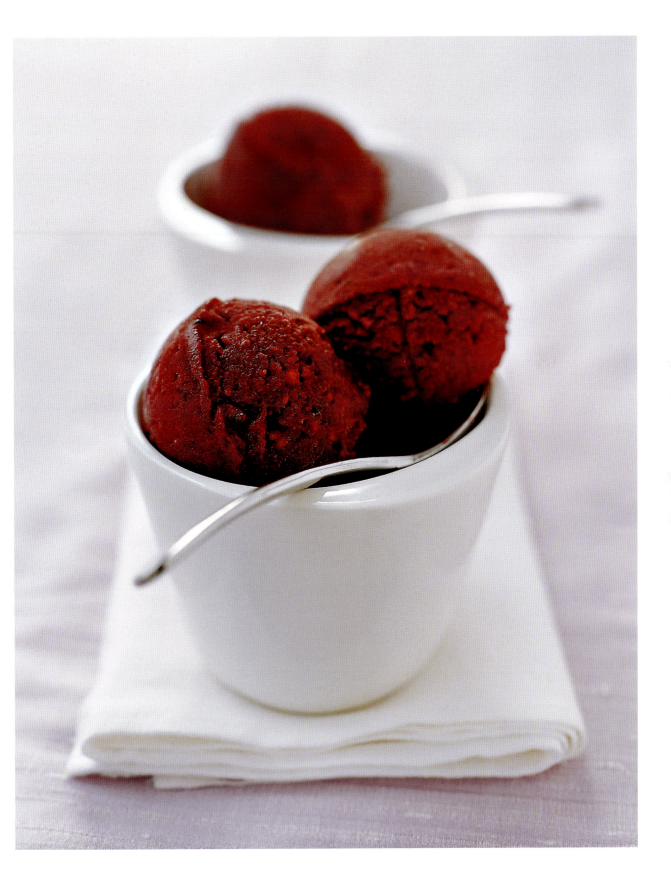

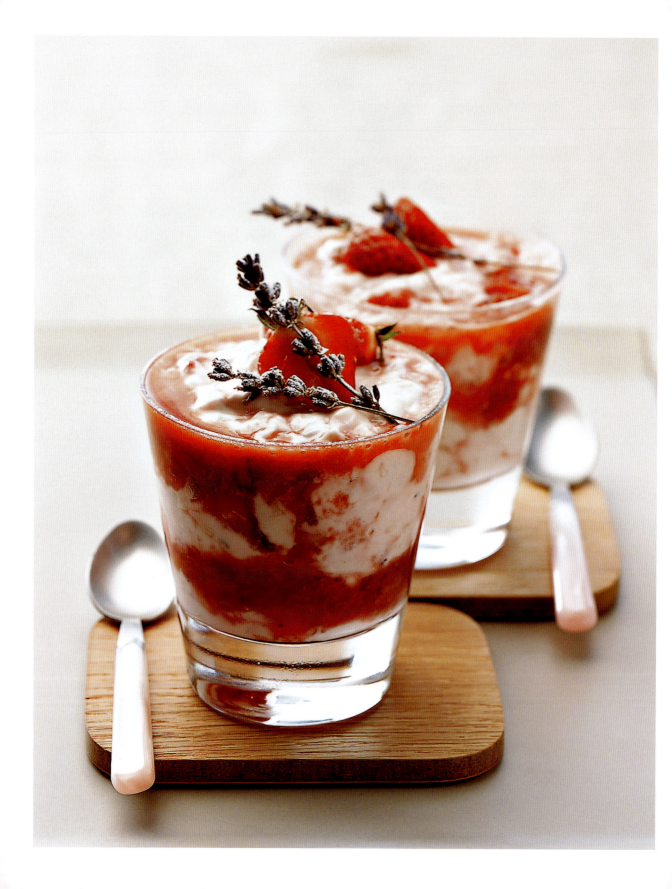

SERVES 4

PREPARATION TIME 10 MINUTES

> Hazelnuts are a top source of the antioxidant vitamin E, which protects cells from damage and enhances the immune system.

strawberry & lavender crush

400 g (13 oz) fresh strawberries

2 tablespoons icing sugar, plus extra for dusting

4–5 lavender flower stems, plus extra to decorate

400 ml (14 fl oz) Greek-style yogurt

100 g (3½ oz) chopped hazelnuts

Reserve 4 small strawberries for decoration. Hull the remainder, put in a bowl with the icing sugar and mash together with a fork. Alternatively, process the strawberries and icing sugar in a food processor or blender to a smooth purée. Pull off the lavender flowers from the stems and crumble them into the purée to taste.

Put the yogurt in a bowl, crumble in the hazelnuts, then lightly mix together. Add the strawberry purée and fold together with a spoon until marbled. Spoon into 4 dessert glasses.

Cut the reserved strawberries in half, then use to decorate the desserts, together with the lavender flowers. Lightly dust with icing sugar and serve immediately.

FOR PEACH & ROSEWATER CRUSH

Peel, halve and stone 3 peaches, then roughly chop and mash or process in a food processor or blender with 2 tablespoons clear honey and 2 teaspoons rosewater. Continue with the recipe as above, but decorate the desserts with crystallized rose petals.

MAKES 14

PREPARATION TIME 20 MINUTES

COOKING TIME 15 MINUTES

Some studies suggest ginger can decrease levels of inflammation, especially in the joints.

stem ginger & dark choc cookies

6 tablespoons golden syrup

50 g (2 oz) vegan spread

115 g (4 oz) rolled oats

75 g (3 oz) wholemeal plain flour

1 teaspoon baking powder

50 g (2 oz) well-drained stem ginger in syrup, finely chopped

50 g (2 oz) plain dark chocolate (70% cocoa solids), roughly chopped

Heat the golden syrup and vegan spread in a small saucepan over a gentle heat until melted, stirring. Allow to cool slightly.

Mix all the remaining ingredients together in a large bowl. Pour in the syrup mixture and mix to form a soft dough. Place 14 spoonfuls of the mixture well spaced apart on a large baking sheet lined with baking paper and gently press with the back of a spoon to flatten slightly. Bake in a preheated oven, 180°C (350°F), Gas Mark 4, for 8–10 minutes until pale golden.

Leave the cookies to cool on the baking sheet for 5 minutes until firm, then transfer to a wire rack to cool completely.

FOR SPICED HAZELNUT & RAISIN COOKIES

Melt the golden syrup and vegan spread as above. Mix together 75 g (3 oz) each rolled oats, wholemeal plain flour and raisins, 50 g (2 oz) lightly toasted and chopped hazelnuts and 1 teaspoon each baking powder and mixed spice in a large bowl. Pour in the syrup mixture and mix to form a soft dough. Continue with the recipe above to form, bake and cool the cookies.

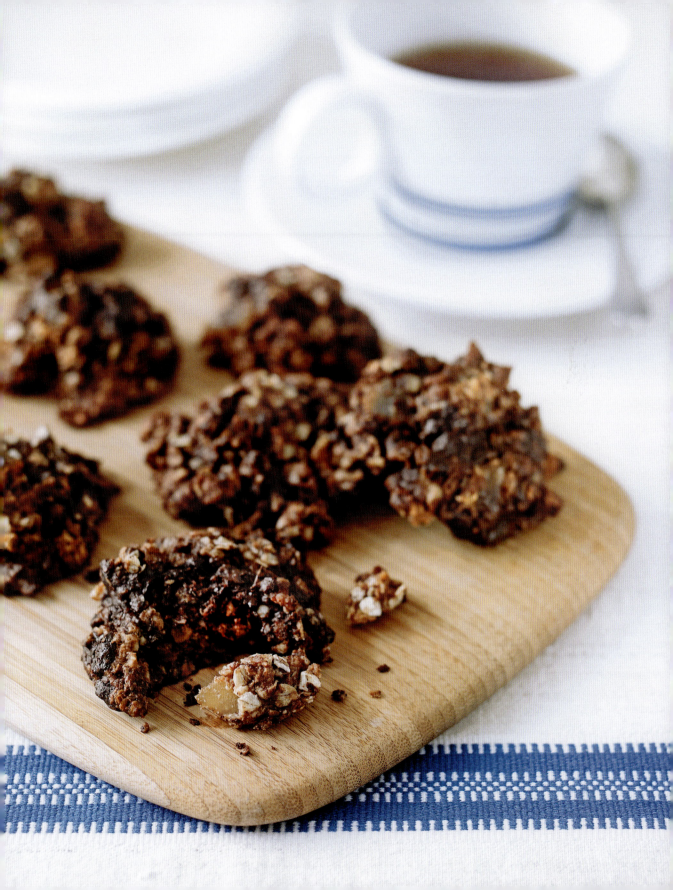

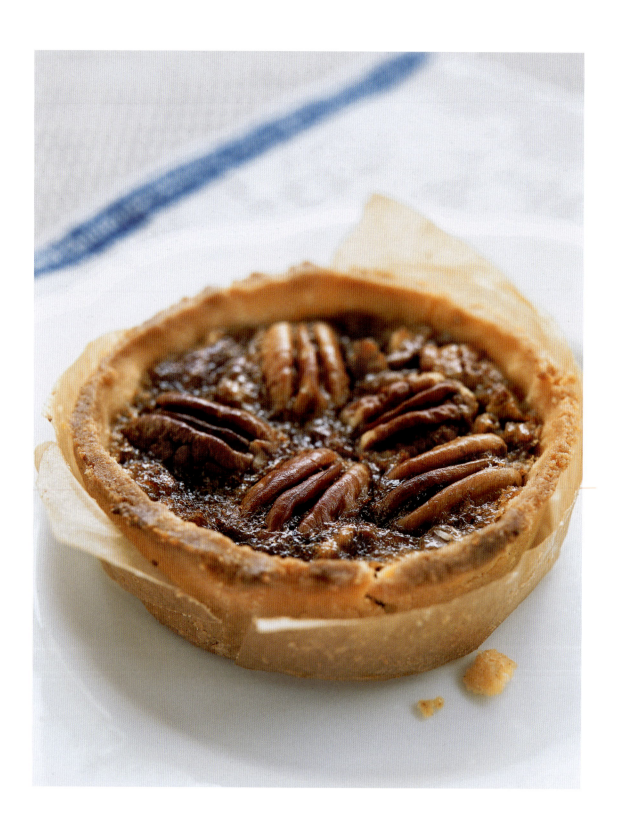

MAKES 8
PREPARATION TIME 15 MINUTES, PLUS CHILLING
COOKING TIME 20–25 MINUTES

Pecans provide lots of manganese, an antioxidant which helps maintain bones and connective tissues.

perfect pecan pies

75 g (3 oz) brown rice flour, plus extra for dusting

50 g (2 oz) chickpea flour

75 g (3 oz) polenta

1 teaspoon xanthan gum

125 g (4 oz) butter, cubed

2 tablespoons caster sugar

1 egg, beaten

FILLING

100 g (3½ oz) soft light brown sugar

150 g (5 oz) butter

125 g (4 oz) honey

175 g (6 oz) pecan nut halves, half roughly chopped

2 eggs, beaten

Grease and line 8 individual 11.5 cm (4½ inch) pie tins. Place the flours, polenta, xanthan gum and butter in a food processor and whizz until the mixture resembles fine breadcrumbs. Alternatively, mix together the flours, polenta and xanthan gum in a large bowl. Add the butter and rub in with the fingertips until the mixture resembles fine breadcrumbs. Stir in the sugar.

Add the egg and enough cold water to form a dough. Knead for a couple of minutes, then wrap in clingfilm and chill for about 1 hour.

Place the sugar, butter and honey for the filling in a saucepan and heat until the sugar has dissolved. Leave to cool for 10 minutes.

Turn the dough out on a surface lightly dusted with rice flour and knead to soften it a little. Divide the dough into 8, then roll each piece out to a thickness of 2.5 mm (1/8 inch) and use to line the pie tins. Stir the chopped pecans and eggs into the filling mixture and pour into the pastry-lined tins. Arrange the pecan halves on top.

Bake in a preheated oven, 200°C (400°F), Gas Mark 6, for 15–20 minutes until the filling is firm. Leave to cool in the tins.

FOR HOMEMADE VANILLA ICE CREAM, TO SERVE AS AN ACCOMPANIMENT

Whip 300 ml (½ pint) double cream with 2 tablespoons caster sugar in a bowl until it forms soft peaks. Fold in a 400 g (13 oz) can ready-made custard and 1 teaspoon vanilla extract. Pour into a freezer-proof container and freeze for 2 hours, then stir with a fork. Put back in the freezer for at least 6 hours, or until solid, then serve with the pecan pies.

SERVES 8
PREPARATION TIME 15 MINUTES
COOKING TIME 20 MINUTES

chocolate & chestnut roulade

butter, for greasing

6 eggs, separated

125 g (4 oz) caster sugar

2 tablespoons cocoa powder

icing sugar, for dusting

FILLING

150 ml (¼ pint) double cream

100 g (3½ oz) chestnut purée or sweetened chestnut spread

Grease and line a 29 x 18 cm (11½ x 7 inch) Swiss roll tin.

Whisk the egg whites in a large clean bowl until they form soft peaks. Whisk together the egg yolks and sugar in a separate bowl until thick and pale. Fold the cocoa powder and egg whites into the egg yolk mixture.

Spoon the mixture into the prepared tin and place in a preheated oven, 180°C (350°F), Gas Mark 4, for 20 minutes. Remove from the oven and leave to cool in the tin.

Turn the cooled sponge out on to a piece of greaseproof paper dusted with icing sugar.

Whip the cream for the filling in a large clean bowl until it forms soft peaks. Fold the chestnut purée or sweetened chestnut spread into the cream, then smooth the filling over the sponge.

Using the greaseproof paper to help you, carefully roll up the roulade from one short end and lift it gently on to its serving dish. (Don't worry if it cracks: it won't detract from its appearance or taste.) Dust with icing sugar. Chill until needed and eat on the day it is made.

FOR CHOCOLATE & BLACK CHERRY ROULADE

Make the sponge as above. To make the filling, omit the chestnut purée or spread and replace it with a 400 g (13 oz) can drained black cherries. Spread over the sponge, roll up and dust with icing sugar.

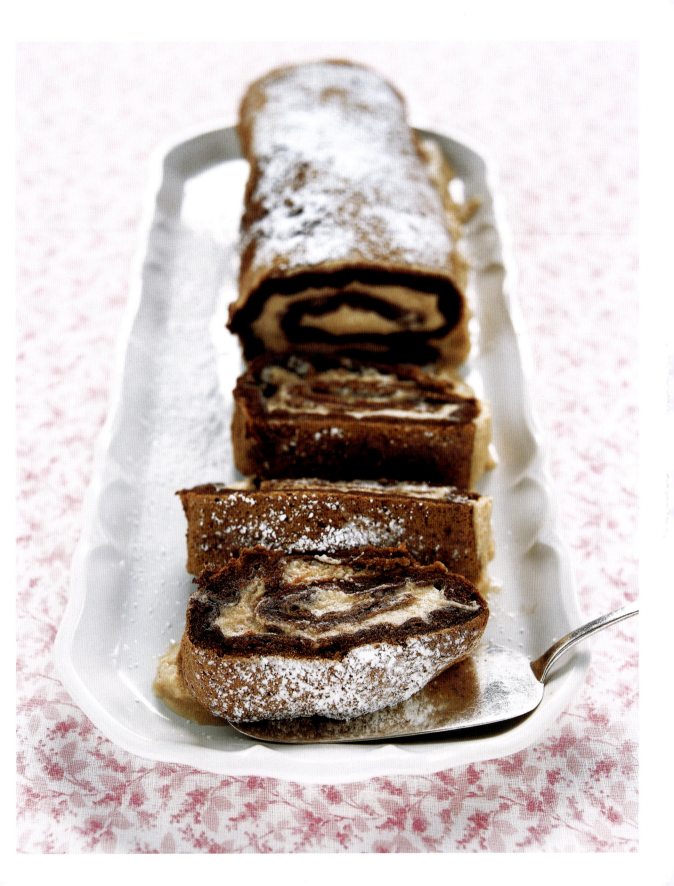

Index

almonds 61, 146, 205
apricots 61
asparagus & goats' cheese risotto 122
asparagus with sesame dressing 189
asparagus, mint & lemon risotto 122
aubergines
    aubergine bake 150
    aubergine dip with flatbreads 109
    aubergine, chilli & chicken bake 150
    spicy aubergine pasta with pine nuts 153
avocado 83
    guacamole with pickled ginger 90

bananas 36
    banana muffins 29
    banana, blueberry & wheatgerm muffins 29
basil 31
    basil oil 105
beans 77
    bean, lemon & rosemary hummus 116
    broad beans with mint & lemon 185
    cannellini & green bean salad 54
    Mediterranean-style beans 39
    mixed bean goulash 39
    mixed bean salad 77
    Niçoise salad 85
    smashed bean & sardine dip 117
    tomato & bean salad 78
    white bean & tomato salad 54
beef
    roast beef & wholegrain mustard potato salad 57
beetroot 106, 113
    beetroot & orange salad 81
berries 29
    mixed berry salad 206
    summer berry sorbet 210
    warm berry salad 206
blackcurrant & almond yogurt 205
bread
    cheat's Mediterranean focaccia 101
    home-baked seeded rolls 24
    mixed seed loaf 24
broccoli 129
bruschetta with fig, rocket & feta 105
bruschetta with tomatoes & ricotta 105
bulgur wheat salad 144
butternut squash
    butternut & cumin soup 166
    butternut squash risotto cakes 168
    roasted butternut & cumin salad 166
    roasted butternut squash risotto 138

cardamom 197
carrot & cashew nut salad 65
carrot & celeriac coleslaw 65
cheese 26, 180
    asparagus & goats' cheese risotto 122
    bruschetta with fig, rocket & feta 105
    bruschetta with tomatoes & ricotta 105
    chickpea & feta salad 69
    courgette, beetroot & feta fritters 113
    Florentine-style eggs 45
    Mediterranean-style vegetable pie 130
    olive, feta & herb scones 41
    pumpkin, feta & pine nut salad 50
    ricotta-stuffed mushrooms 110
    spinach, potato & ricotta frittata 38
    spinach, tomato & Parmesan scones 41
    watermelon & halloumi salad 69
    watermelon, feta & herb salad 62
cherries
    chocolate & black cherry roulade 218
chestnut purée 218
chicken
    aubergine, chilli & chicken bake 150
    chargrilled chicken with salsa & fruity couscous 128
    chicken bites with salsa 114
    chicken couscous salad 82
    chicken, apricot & almond

salad 61
chicken, lemon & olive stew 142
creamy paprika chicken 133
creamy pesto chicken with lemon 133
grilled chicken with apricot & tomato salad 61
Mediterranean olive chicken 157
polenta crusted chicken 149
spiced chicken & mango salad 83
sun-dried tomato & chicken couscous 128
sweet chilli chicken patties 165
Thai-style chicken soup 169
chickpeas
  chickpea & chilli hummus 116
  chickpea & feta salad 69
  chickpea falafel 98
  harissa & tahini hummus 102
  Moroccan pan-roasted chickpeas 102
chillies 59, 116, 150, 153
  chilli prawn, mango & avocado salad 83
  chilli, lime & coriander dried fruit & nuts 93
chocolate 214
  chewy nutty chocolate brownies 202
  chocolate & black cherry roulade 218
  chocolate & chestnut roulade 218
  chocolate & orange mousse 209
  rich chocolate mousse 209
chorizo & potato omelette 46
ciabatta toasties with Mediterranean vegetables 174
clementines 201
coriander 93
courgette, beetroot & feta fritters 113
couscous
  chargrilled chicken with salsa & fruity couscous 128
  chicken couscous salad 82
  sun-dried tomato & chicken couscous 128
crème fraîche
  creamy paprika chicken 133
  creamy pesto chicken with lemon 133
cress 23
cucumber
  cucumber & mint dip 109
  cucumber & yogurt dip 113
  Greek-style salad 74
  pickled cucumber & chilli salad 59
cumin seeds 166

eggs 23, 35, 38
  Florentine-style eggs 45
  herby smoked salmon omelettes 22
  Niçoise salad 85
  omelette with basil tomatoes 31
  pesto scrambled eggs 32
  poached eggs & spinach 23
  rice & sweetcorn omelette 46
  smoked ham & tomato omelette 22
  spinach, potato & ricotta frittata 38
  tomato-stuffed omelette 31
fennel & salmon soup 125
figs 105
  fig & honey pots 198
  fig, bean & toasted pecan salad 77
  hot figs with honey 198

fish pie 154
fruit 62, 93, 128, 194
  autumn fruit oaty crumble 201
  forest fruit & clementine crumble 201
  fruit granola bars 36
  traditional fruit cake 194
  tropical fruit cake 194
  vanilla-spiced fruit salad 199

garlic 180
  garlic & tomato seafood spaghetti 145
  Greek-style salad with garlic pitta bread 74
ginger 90, 173, 181
  gingered tofu & mango salad 73
  stem ginger & dark choc cookies 214
granola bars 36
granola with peaches & yogurt 21
guacamole with pickled ginger 90

ham
  smoked ham & tomato omelette 22
harissa 118
  harissa & tahini hummus 102
hazelnuts 36
  spiced hazelnut & raisin cookies 214
herbs 41, 62
  herb oatcakes 96
  herby smoked salmon omelettes 22
honey 198
  honeyed pumpkin & ginger broth 173

ice cream
  homemade vanilla ice cream 217

lavender 213
lemons 116, 122, 133, 142, 185, 190
   lemony prawns & broccoli stir-fry 129
lentils
   lentil Bolognese 137
   no-cook lentil, tomato & onion salad 70
   spiced green lentils with tomatoes 181
   warm lentil, tomato & onion salad 70
limes 93

mackerel 134
   black pepper & bay mackerel 134
   smoked mackerel crostini 97
   smoked mackerel fishcakes 97
mango 83
   creamy mango & passion fruit 205
   gingered tofu & mango salad 73
mint 98, 109, 122, 141, 185
   minted yogurt 144
muesli, homemade 42
   Bircher muesli 42
mushrooms
   mushroom risotto cakes 168
   pepper & mushroom 'paella' with pine nuts 146
   ricotta-stuffed mushrooms 110
   wild mushroom risotto 138
mustard 57, 180

noodles 126
   prawn & broccoli noodles 129
nuts 65, 93
   chewy nutty chocolate brownies 202

oats 201
   herb oatcakes 96
olive oil 89
olives 142
   cheat's Mediterranean focaccia 101
   green olives with tomatoes & preserved lemon 190
   Mediterranean olive chicken 157
   Niçoise salad 85
   olive, feta & herb scones 41
   sweet potatoes with green olives 190
onions 70
oranges 81, 209
   orange & cardamom rice pudding 197

pak choi 126, 161
parsnip & beetroot crisps with homemade dukkah 106
passion fruit 205
pasta
   garlic & tomato seafood spaghetti 145
   Mediterranean pasta salad 53, 66
   spicy Mediterranean pasta 153
   vegetable spaghetti Bolognese 137
peaches 21
   peach & rosewater crush 213
pear, banana & hazelnut granola bars 36
peas
   pea & mint falafel with mint dip 98
   pea & pesto soup 182
   tofu & sugar snap salad 73
   yellow split peas with tomatoes & ginger 181
pecan nuts 77
   perfect pecan pies 217
peppers 38
   baby green peppers in olive oil 89
   charred green pepper toasts 89
   pepper & mushroom 'paella' with pine nuts 146
pesto, homemade 32, 133, 182
   pesto scrambled eggs 32
pine nuts 50, 146, 153
polenta crusted chicken 149
pomegranate vinaigrette 82
potatoes 38, 46, 57, 177
   Mediterranean potato salad 66
   Niçoise salad 85
   potato rösti with frazzled eggs 35
   rösti with poached eggs 35
   rösti-topped fish pie 154
prawns 83, 129
   prawn & broccoli noodles 129
pumpkin 173
   pumpkin, feta & pine nut salad 50
   roasted spiced pumpkin 186

quinoa
   turkey balls with minty quinoa 141

raisins 214
raspberry sorbet 210
rice 168, 197
   asparagus, mint & lemon risotto 122
   butternut squash risotto cakes 168
   Mediterranean rice salad 53
   rice & sweetcorn omelette 46
   rice pudding 197

roasted butternut squash risotto 138
wild mushroom risotto 138
rocket 105
rosewater 213

salmon 22, 125
- crusted salmon with tomato salsa 149
- roasted salmon & vegetables 125
- smoked salmon & potato salad 57
sardines 117
seafood
- garlic & tomato seafood spaghetti 145
sesame seeds 189
spices 106, 133, 170, 186
- spiced hazelnut & raisin cookies 214
- spiced mackerel fillets 134
- spiced tofu, noodles & pak choi 126
spinach 23
- spinach & fish pie 154
- spinach, egg & cress salad 23
- spinach, potato & ricotta frittata 38
- spinach, tomato & Parmesan scones 41
- sweet spinach 142
strawberry & lavender crush 213
sweet chilli sauce
- sweet chilli chicken patties 165
- sweet chilli vegetable stir-fry 161
sweet potato & garlic mash 180
sweet potato, cheese & mustard mash 180
sweet potatoes with green olives 190

sweetcorn 46
- sweetcorn & roasted pepper frittata 38

tahini 102
tofu 73
- baked teriyaki tofu bites 94
- spiced tofu, noodles & pak choi 126
- stir-fried tofu with hoisin sauce 126
- tandoori tofu bites 94
- tofu & sugar snap salad 73
tomatoes 22, 31, 41, 54, 61, 70, 105, 145, 149, 181, 190
- Greek-style salad 74
- Mediterranean-style tomato soup 162
- Niçoise salad 85
- panzanella-style salad 78
- sun-dried tomato & chicken couscous 128
- tomato & bean salad 78
- tomato-stuffed omelette 31
tortillas 109, 177
- chicken bites with salsa 114
tuna 170
- spiced tuna open sandwiches 170
- spicy tuna wraps 177
- tuna & jalapeño baked potatoes 177
- tuna Niçoise salad 85
turkey
- minced turkey salad 58
- turkey & cheese sandwiches 26
- turkey balls with minty quinoa 141
- turkey croque madame 26

vegetables 125, 161, 174
- baby leaf stir-fry with chilli 165
- baby vegetables with pesto 182
- Mediterranean-style vegetable pie 130
- mixed pickled vegetables 178
- pickled vegetable salad 59
- vegetable 'paella' with almonds 146
- vegetable kebabs with harissa yogurt 118
- vegetable spaghetti Bolognese 137
- veggie kebabs with bulgur wheat 144
- veggie stir-fry with pak choi 161

watermelon & halloumi salad 69
watermelon fruit salad 62
watermelon, feta & herb salad 62

yogurt 21, 113, 118, 144
- blackcurrant & almond yogurt 205
- creamy mango & passion fruit 205

UK–US Glossary

UK	US
Aubergine	Eggplant
Baking paper	Baking parchment
Beetroot	Beet
Bicarbonate of soda	Baking soda
Butter beans	Lima beans
Celeriac	Celery root
Chestnut mushrooms	Cremini mushrooms
Clingfilm	Plastic wrap
Coriander (fresh)	Cilantro
Cornflour	Cornstarch
Courgette	Zucchini
Cream, single/double	Cream, light/heavy
Desiccated coconut	Shredded dried coconut
Dried chilli flakes	Crushed red pepper flakes
Flaked almonds	Slivered almonds
Flour, plain/self-raising	Flour, all-purpose/self-rising
Foil	Aluminium foil
Frying pan	Skillet
Grated	Shredded
Grill	Broil
Ground almonds	Almond meal
Jug	Pitcher
Kitchen paper	Paper towel
Mangetout	Snow peas
Minced turkey	Ground turkey
Mixed spice	Pie spice mix
Natural yogurt	Plain yogurt
Pak choi	Boy choy
Pepper (red)	Bell pepper
Plain dark chocolate	Semi-sweet chocolate
Polenta	Cornmeal
Prawns	Shrimp
Rapeseed oil	Canola oil
Rocket	Arugula
Spring onion	Scallion
Stock	Broth
Sugar, caster/icing	Sugar, superfine/confectioners'
Sultanas	Golden raisins
Tea towel	Cloth kitchen towel
Tomato purée	Tomato paste

Picture Credits

Octopus Publishing Group: Frank Adam 52; Stephen Conroy 131, 175; Will Heap 92, 107, 119, 152, 172, 179, 187; David Munns 135, 164; Lis Parsons 6, 51, 56, 60, 72, 75, 79, 80, 84, 115, 143, 163, 171, 207; William Shaw 7, 11, 20, 25, 27, 28, 37, 40, 43, 44, 47, 55, 63, 64, 68, 71, 76, 88, 91, 95, 99, 100, 103, 111, 112, 123, 124, 127, 132, 136, 139, 140, 147, 148, 151, 155, 156, 160, 167, 176, 183, 184, 188, 191, 195, 196, 200, 203, 204, 215, 216, 219; Ian Wallace 5, 9, 33, 34, 67, 104, 108, 208, 211, 212.